**PHYSICAL
FITNESS**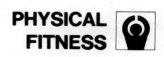

Other Preventive Medicine Institute/Strang Clinic
HEALTH ACTION PLANS

 How to Stop Smoking

 Nutrition

 Personal and Family Safety and Crime Prevention

PHYSICAL FITNESS

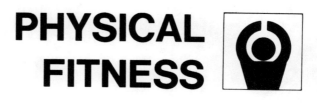

A Preventive Medicine Institute/Strang Clinic
HEALTH ACTION PLAN

MARILYN SNYDER HALPER, M.P.H.
IRA NEIGER

Series Editor
Daniel G. Miller, M.D.

Associate Editors
Bernard Gutin, Ph.D.
Anne Marie Kelly
Pamela Hatch

Holt, Rinehart and Winston   New York

Copyright © 1980 by Preventive Medicine Institute/Strang Clinic

All rights reserved, including the right to reproduce
this book or portions thereof in any form.

First published in January 1981 by Holt, Rinehart and Winston,
383 Madison Avenue, New York, New York 10017.

Published simultaneously in Canada by Holt, Rinehart and
Winston of Canada, Limited.

Library of Congress Cataloging in Publication Data

Halper, Marilyn Snyder.
    Physical fitness.

    (A Preventive Medicine Institute/Strang Clinic
health action plan)
    Includes index.
    1. Physical fitness. 2. Exercise. I. Neiger,
Ira, joint author. II. Title. III. Series: Pre-
ventive Medicine Institute/Strang Clinic. Preventive
Medicine Institute/Strang Clinic health action plan.
RA781.H34   613.7   80-10847

ISBN Hardbound: 0-03-048291-7
ISBN Paperback: 0-03-048286-0

First Edition

Designer: Betty Binns Graphics
Printed in the United States of America
10 9 8 7 6 5 4 3 2 1

Contents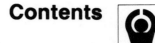

Part 6
SPECIAL PROGRAMS

Part 7
A FEW FINAL THOUGHTS

Foreword

After more than four years of research, study, and testing, it is with great pride and pleasure that we bring you this Preventive Medicine Institute/Strang Clinic Health Action Plan. The development of this book (one of four currently available) has been one of the most exciting—and, we believe, successful—projects the clinic has ever undertaken. By making use of the Health Action Plans, you will be taking a major step toward improving your own health as well as that of your family.

Taken together, these plans address the health problems—cancer, heart disease, and accidents—responsible for the majority of chronic illnesses, disabilities, and premature deaths in this country. The four books—*Personal and Family Safety, How to Stop Smoking, Nutrition,* and *Physical Fitness*—deal directly with the behaviors most closely associated with these health concerns.

Until recently, it has been generally assumed that advanced technology, more physicians, and better medical care would ensure the health and increase the life spans of most Americans. While we have made tremendous progress in the fields of disease detection and cure, and life expectancy has increased dramatically since the turn of the century, considerable evidence indicates that we have reached a point of diminishing returns. Life expectancy has leveled off in the last few decades, and disease patterns have changed. Infectious diseases such as tuberculosis, pneumonia, and typhoid, once among the most feared health problems, have, for the most part, been replaced by chronic disorders such as cancer and heart disease.

The path to the control of chronic diseases lies in a new direction. While we don't have all the answers, we do have hard evidence that links cancer to smoking, implicates high-fat diets and obesity in cancer and heart disease, and suggests that lack of regular exercise contributes to heart and respiratory problems.

To put it another way, the major causes of chronic disease, disability, and death in the Western world have one important thing in common: they are all connected to some extent to our behavior, our habits. Improved health, therefore, unquestionably will depend upon our ability to throw away our cigarettes, change our dietary habits, exercise regularly, and learn to take precautions against avoidable accidents. In today's world, health depends more on our ability to *prevent* diseases and accidents than on our ability to treat their effects once they have occurred. And since the decision to live wisely is an individual's choice, your health, to a great extent, is in your own hands.

Our belief in the concept of preventive medicine led us to develop the Health Action Plans. Many reputable books on related subjects are available, but we believe ours are unique for three reasons. First, their ultimate objective is *permanent* change in everyday health habits and life-styles. Second, each Health Action Plan provides a *structured* approach to behavioral change—a simple, step-by-step way to achieve personal health-related goals. Third, the structure is similar in each of the Health Action Plans, so if you use one, you will find the format of the others familiar, allowing you to readily develop your own *individualized and integrated* programs.

Each book includes a section on self-assessment to give you a deeper understanding of your current habits. Once you have been made aware of the details of these habits, you are given suggestions for making health-improving changes as well as the tools for achieving your specific goals. In addition, each book makes provision for maintaining change once it has been achieved. The maintenance plans often involve record keeping, which not only increases your awareness and knowledge of a health habit, but arms you with additional reinforcement for further change.

All the Health Action Plans were developed with the help of consultants and consumers. People like you were asked to test each plan and to make suggestions. These consumers were discriminating critics, and their contributions benefited the plans greatly. Health consultants—doctors, nutritionists, exercise physiologists, and other experts—have also carefully considered each program, commenting on content and accuracy and helping in program testing.

None of these plans provides an instant answer: rather, they are personally focused programs for modifying the way you live so that you and your family can enjoy long, happy—and healthy lives.

A person's health must ultimately be his or her own responsibility. We hope that these Health Action Plans will provide you with a practical and reliable guide to a healthier life.

Daniel G. Miller, M.D.
Director, Preventive Medicine
Institute/Strang Clinic

A word about the Preventive Medicine Institute/Strang Clinic

The Preventive Medicine Institute/Strang Clinic is a nonprofit organization dedicated to the prevention of cancer, heart disease, stroke, and other serious illnesses. Established at Memorial Hospital in New York City in 1940 by Dr. Elise Strang L'Esperance, the Strang Clinic originally became well known for its pioneering use of the Pap test, the screening technique for cervical cancer devised by Dr. George Papanicolaou. In 1963 the clinic became an independent center. At that time the clinic—which until then had been devoted largely to cancer detection—broadened its scope to cover diagnosis, research, and detection of all the major chronic and controllable diseases. In 1966 the clinic was renamed the Preventive Medicine Institute/Strang Clinic, with the Strang Clinic serving as the clinical division and the institute serving as the research center.

During the past ten years, the focus of the clinic's work has again widened, emphasizing health education and the role of the individual in preventing disease. In this respect, its goal has been to devise lifelong health and safety programs that deter the onset of disease and injury.

Acknowledgments

The Preventive Medicine Institute/Strang Clinic staff would like to thank the following consultants for their assistance and valuable suggestions:

Bernard Gutin, Ph.D.
Exercise Physiologist
Teachers College
Columbia University

Charles A. Bucher, Ph.D.
Professor of Education
Director
School of Education, Health,
  Nursing and Arts Professions
New York University
Department of Physical Education
  and Sport

Paul Vallario, M.A.
Doctoral Candidate, New York University
Physical Fitness and Health Consultant

We also wish to acknowledge the contributions of Sandra Gagliardo for her resource gathering and Wendy Seda and Petra Vera of Preventive Medicine Institute/Strang Clinic for their assistance.

Introduction

With so many books about physical fitness and exercise already on the market, you are probably asking yourself, What makes this book different? How is this book unique? If you have picked up this book, you are probably already motivated to start a fitness program, but you may be a bit bewildered about how to establish an effective program or about precisely what you should expect to achieve through exercising.

The Health Action Plan, *Physical Fitness,* is unique in that, unlike other programs, it will help you to identify your personal reasons for wanting to establish a regular fitness program, and, as a result, it will enable you to begin to construct goals to meet your needs. In addition, the Health Action Plan tells you how to design a personal exercise regimen to suit your special goals, needs, and requirements. Finally, because maintenance is important for long-term gain in any fitness program, this plan provides you with tools for assuring that you will keep up your fitness activity. The basic fitness program is designed, with an eye toward safety and individual suitability, for all healthy adults.

In addition to "The Basic Health Action Plan for Physical Fitness," we have also designed programs to meet special needs. Two moderate fitness programs— an exercise program and a walking program—are useful for older or extremely sedentary people. Several programs for relaxation and tension relief are outlined for those with needs in that area; a lower-back pain program is provided for those with this problem or for those who especially wish to concentrate on that potential problem area.

☐ How to use this book

Before beginning to plan your fitness program, take the three self-assessment tests in Part 1. The purpose of these tests is to identify your reasons for wanting to be fit and thus help you set personal goals for yourself. After taking the tests, summarize your answers on the "Profile Record," pages 10–11. This record will sum up, at a glance, your attitudes toward exercise, your present rate of activity, and your reasons for wanting to exercise. You may be surprised by the results! But more important, you will be able to devise a regimen that will best suit your needs.

Part 2, "Preparing for Fitness," is central to the Health Action Plan, *Physical Fitness,* and should be read with great care. It will provide you with suggestions for making your everyday life more active, which is as important to general physical fitness as a prescribed exercise program. Second, it will teach you how to monitor your pulse rate during vigorous exercise—a pivotal factor in determining your proper rate of progress toward physical fitness.

Part 3, "Putting It All Together," provides you with the tools for devising a personal health action plan. Read the sections on "General Principles About Exercising" and "The Basic Health Action Plan for Physical Fitness" carefully. Then, using the "Guide to Planning Your Fitness Program" as an outline, select exercises from Part 4, "Health Action Plan Exercises," that best suit your tastes, needs, and opportunities. You will notice that few of the exercises require equipment or gadgets, which relieves you of unnecessary expense and enables you to exercise in virtually any setting.

If you are older or have been extremely sedentary, you may wish to start out with one of the moderate fitness programs found in Part 5. Either the exercise program or the walking program will provide you with sufficient exercise to achieve fitness; however, if you wish to graduate to the more vigorous basic program, you can do so once you have mastered the moderate program. It is also strongly suggested that you check with a doctor first.

For those who wish to concentrate on tension relief, you can adapt one of the "Programs for Relaxation and Relief of Tension" into your basic fitness program. For those with back pain, you may wish to use the "Lower-Back Pain Prevention and Relief Program" as your primary exercise regimen or alternate this program with a basic Health Action Plan program.

The Health Action Plan, *Physical Fitness,* has been carefully tested by consumers. Their suggestions were helpful to us in devising these programs, and so we pass their tips on to you. You should find these useful and illuminating as you work up your own fitness program.

We sincerely hope that you will find the Health Action Plan, *Physical Fitness,* helpful as you devise and maintain a program of activity. Good luck!

Part 1

Self-assessment

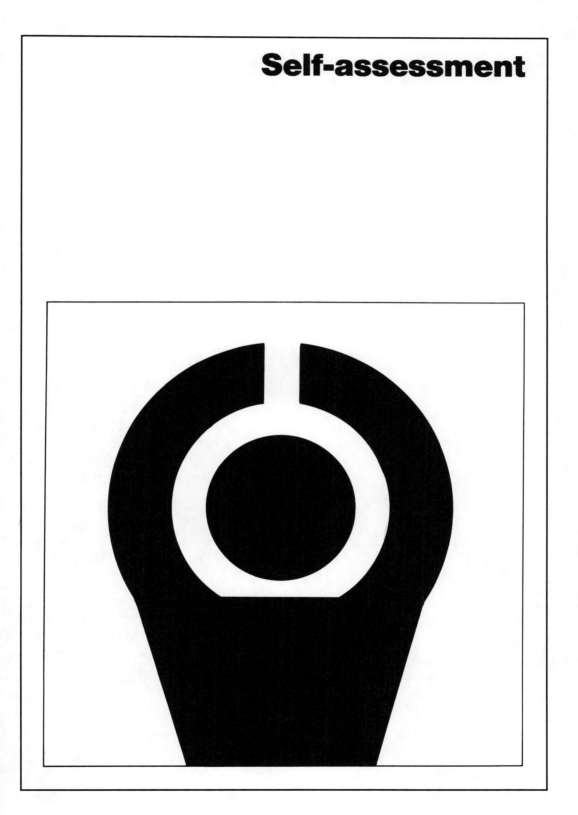

CHAPTER 1
Self-assessment: introduction

The purpose of these tests is to provide you with a clear picture of your attitudes toward exercise. They will help you decide precisely why you want to begin a physical fitness program, what you expect from a program, and how motivated you really are. The tests will help you establish clear goals, guide you toward a program suited to your needs, and give you insight into your ultimate success.

There are three tests in this section. Self-Assessment 1 will help you define and clarify your attitude toward exercise, 2 will help you pinpoint your present level of physical activity, and 3 will help you define your specific goals.

Answer each question on each test. Record your scores and review "How to Interpret Your Scores." Finally, record your scores on the "Profile Record" located on pages 10–11. The completed "Profile Record" will provide you with a summary of results and be a convenient reference as you proceed to create your individual exercise program.

Self-assessment 1
WHAT IS YOUR ATTITUDE TOWARD EXERCISE?

After reading each statement, circle the number that most accurately indicates how you feel. For example, in question ''a,'' if you strongly agree, circle ''1,'' if you agree, circle ''2,'' and so on. Be sure to answer every question.

	Strongly agree	Agree	Disagree	Strongly disagree
a Basically I am a sedentary (inactive) person.	1	2	3	4
b Exercise is enjoyable.	4	3	2	1
c When I was a child, my family encouraged me to exercise.	4	3	2	1
d Exercise is boring.	1	2	3	4
e The ability to master a fitness program would be an exciting challenge to me.	4	3	2	1
f I avoid physical activity.	1	2	3	4
g I have an increased sense of well-being after I exercise vigorously.	4	3	2	1
h I usually find excuses not to exercise.	1	2	3	4
i Maintaining a physical fitness program would show that I have willpower.	4	3	2	1
j Looking good is very important to me.	4	3	2	1
k Physically fit people always look better.	4	3	2	1
l I don't like looking unfit.	4	3	2	1

How to score

Enter the numbers you have circled in answer to questions in Self-Assessment 1 in the appropriate spaces below. Put the number you have circled in question "a" over line "a," the number for question "b" over line "b," and so on. Add the scores across and record the total. For example, the sum of your scores over lines "a," "c," and "f" gives your total score for "Image."

After you have added up your scores, read "How to Interpret Your Scores" and enter your scores on the "Profile Record," page 10.

How to interpret your scores

Scores can vary from 3 to 12. A score of 9 or over is high. A score of 6 or under is low. A score of 7 or 8 is average.

IMAGE

If you scored 9 or more on "Image," you probably think of yourself as a fairly active person. Applying this positive image toward your exercise program will contribute to your success.

If you scored 6 or less, you may be hampered by a negative image of yourself. A sedentary image is often inherited from one's family. A regular fitness program will help you improve that image.

ENJOYMENT

If you scored 9 or more, you already enjoy exercise. This ability will help you maintain a regular long-term fitness program.

If you scored 6 or less, you probably do not enjoy exercising. Remember: you can take steps to make exercising more pleasant. Try working out with a friend, exercising to music, or finding a more pleasant location.

APPEARANCE

If you scored 9 or above, your appearance is quite important to you. Your positive attitude with regard to your appearance will help you succeed in establishing an exercise program.

If you scored 6 or below, appearance is not your most important motivation for fitness. But keep in mind that a fit figure is attractive at any age.

DISCIPLINE

If you scored 9 or more, it is important to you to be in control of your life. This attitude will serve as an effective tool in helping you succeed with a regular fitness program.

If you scored 6 or less, making use of the record-keeping charts should be encouraging, and record keeping will aid you in learning to control your daily patterns and habits.

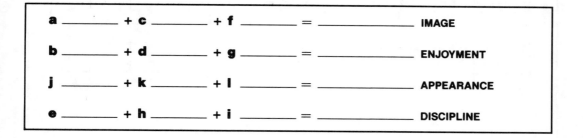

a _____ + c _____ + f _____ = _____ IMAGE

b _____ + d _____ + g _____ = _____ ENJOYMENT

j _____ + k _____ + l _____ = _____ APPEARANCE

e _____ + h _____ + i _____ = _____ DISCIPLINE

Self-assessment 2
WHAT IS YOUR PRESENT LEVEL OF PHYSICAL ACTIVITY?

Read each statement and circle the number that most accurately describes how you feel. For example, in question "a," if you always feel that way, circle "4," if you often do, circle "3," and so on. Be sure to answer every question.

	Always	Often	Sometimes	Never
a I walk rather than ride whenever possible.	4	3	2	1
b I exercise more than once a week.	4	3	2	1
c I don't have enough time to exercise.	1	2	3	4
d I use stairs rather than elevators or escalators.	4	3	2	1
e I have a formal exercise plan that I follow.	4	3	2	1
f I find time every day to do something active.	4	3	2	1
g Most of my workday is spent sitting behind a desk.	1	2	3	4
h I participate in some sport (tennis, dancing, jogging, swimming) at least once a week.	4	3	2	1

How to score

Enter the numbers you have circled in answer to questions in Self-Assessment 2 in the appropriate spaces below. Put the number you have circled in question "a" over line "a," the number for question "b" over line "b," and so on. Add the scores across and record the total. For example, the sum of your scores over lines "b," "c," "e," and "h" gives you your total score for "Exercise."

After you have added up your scores, read "How to Interpret Your Scores" and enter your scores on the "Profile Record," page 11.

How to interpret your scores

Scores can vary from 4 to 16. A score of 12 or over is high. A score of 8 or under is low. A score of 9 to 11 is average.

EXERCISE

If you scored 12 or above, you already exercise fairly regularly and are well on your way to a successful fitness program. You may have to increase your current exercise level only slightly. Look carefully at your goals and remodel your present program to fit them.

If you scored 8 or below, you are probably not exercising enough. Pay close attention to the exercises suggested in this book. They take only a modest amount of time, but if you stick with them, you will be amazed at how much they can do for you.

ACTIVITY

If you scored 12 or above, you lead a fairly active life. You may want to increase the amount of your daily activity and include a regular exercise program. Because you are already active, you are on the right track.

If you scored 8 or below, you are probably an inactive person. You do not tend to think of active ways to do everyday things. Increasing the number of times you walk, climb stairs, and move from place to place each day can improve your body function and prepare you for an exercise program.

COMPOSITE SCORE

Add your total exercise score and your total activity score and you have your composite score. Your composite score will help you select the appropriate level of exercise at which to begin. Enter your total exercise score and your total activity score on your "Profile Record," page 11.

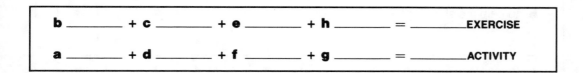

b _____ + c _____ + e _____ + h _____ = _____EXERCISE

a _____ + d _____ + f _____ + g _____ = _____ACTIVITY

Self-assessment 3
WHY DO YOU WANT TO BE PHYSICALLY FIT?

The following are reasons people frequently give to explain why they want to be physically fit and what they hope to gain from a fitness program. Circle the number that best describes your attitude. For example, if you think reason "a" is extremely important, circle "4," if you think it is fairly important, circle "3," and so on. Be sure to answer every question.

	Extremely important	Fairly important	Not very important	Unimportant
a To protect myself from heart problems.	4	3	2	1
b To have more energy.	4	3	2	1
c To increase my work efficiency.	4	3	2	1
d To relieve my feelings of tiredness.	4	3	2	1
e To relieve tension.	4	3	2	1
f To trim my waist.	4	3	2	1
g To streamline my body.	4	3	2	1
h To help me sleep better.	4	3	2	1
i To relieve stress.	4	3	2	1
j To increase my wind capacity.	4	3	2	1
k To eliminate bulges.	4	3	2	1
l To tighten sagging muscles.	4	3	2	1
m To lose weight.	4	3	2	1
n To lower my blood pressure.	4	3	2	1
o To protect myself from injury and accidents.	4	3	2	1

How to score

Enter the numbers you have circled in answer to questions in Self-Assessment 3 in the appropriate spaces below. Put the number you have circled for reason "a" over line "a," the number for reason "b" over line "b," and so on.

Add the scores across and record the total. For example, the sum of your scores over lines "a," "j," and "n" gives you your total score for "Heart Rate and Respiratory Reserve."

After you have added up your scores, read "How to Interpret Your Scores" and enter your scores on the "Profile Record," page 11.

How to interpret your scores

A score of 9 or over means this goal is very important to you. The higher your score, up to 12, the more important the goal.

HEART RATE AND RESPIRATORY RESERVE

If you scored 9 or above, the efficiency of your heart and lungs is very important to you. When making up a fitness program, include exercises that will condition the cardiovascular and respiratory systems.

STRESS AND TENSION RELIEF

If you scored 9 or above, you want an exercise program to help relieve tension and probably help you sleep. Exercises cannot eliminate the stressful situations in your life, but they can provide a release from general tension and improve your ability to relax.

ENERGY

A score of 9 or over indicates that you are not satisfied with your present energy level. Exercise will increase your ability to work and play longer than you are able to now and without getting as tired.

MUSCLE TONE AND GENERAL CONDITIONING

A score of 9 or over means you are concerned with sagging, out-of-shape, or weak muscles. Good muscle tone means not only that your body is in good condition but also that you have added protection from injury and a better appearance. If you scored high, see Chapter 20, "Exercise and Your Appearance."

FAT REDUCTION

A score of 9 or over means you are concerned with excess weight and bulges. If you are overweight, don't forget that exercise alone will not take off enough of the extra pounds. The right course of action is a combination of exercise, which burns calories, and calorie reduction. Certain bulges (hips, thighs) can be trimmed down by exercise. However, exercise cannot change your body type. If you are tall and have a big frame, or if you are small-boned, you will remain that way. But exercise can make your body look its best no matter what type of build you have. If your score was high, see Chapter 20, "Exercise and Your Appearance."

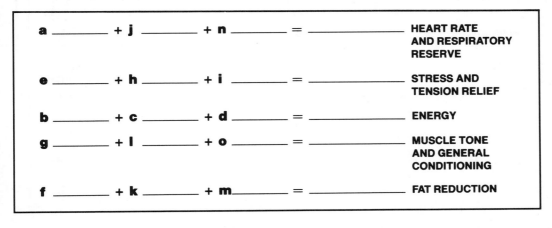

a _____ + j _____ + n _____ = _____			HEART RATE AND RESPIRATORY RESERVE
e _____ + h _____ + i _____ = _____			STRESS AND TENSION RELIEF
b _____ + c _____ + d _____ = _____			ENERGY
g _____ + l _____ + o _____ = _____			MUSCLE TONE AND GENERAL CONDITIONING
f _____ + k _____ + m _____ = _____			FAT REDUCTION

CHAPTER 2
Profile record

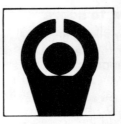

Results of Self-Assessments 1, 2, and 3 should now be completed and entered on your "Profile Record."

Your "Profile Record" can help you assign priorities to determine your most important goals in your exercise program. You should refer to this record throughout your exercise program.

Setting specific and realistic goals for yourself is the most important step you can take toward a successful program, because you will have a standard against which you can measure progress. An important long-term goal is to always include exercise in your everyday life. Long after your specific goals have been met, a successful fitness program will help you remain healthy, trim, and relaxed.

Self-assessment 1
WHAT IS YOUR ATTITUDE TOWARD EXERCISE?

Important attitudes about your exercise habits	Enter your scores from p. 5	Circle if score is 12–10	Circle if score is 9–7	Circle if score is 6–4	Circle if score is 3
		THIS ATTITUDE IS			
IMAGE	_____	Most Important	Important	Somewhat Important	Least Important
ENJOYMENT	_____	Most Important	Important	Somewhat Important	Least Important
APPEARANCE	_____	Most Important	Important	Somewhat Important	Least Important
DISCIPLINE	_____	Most Important	Important	Somewhat Important	Least Important

---

Self-assessment 2
WHAT IS YOUR PRESENT LEVEL OF PHYSICAL ACTIVITY?

How active are you?	Enter your scores from p. 7	Circle if score is 12–10	Circle if score is 9–7	Circle if score is 6–4	Circle if score is 3
		YOUR CURRENT LEVEL IS			
EXERCISE	_____	Very High	High	Moderate	Low
ACTIVITY	_____	Very High	High	Moderate	Low
COMPOSITE SCORE	Total scores of exercise and activity _____				

Self-assessment 3
WHY DO YOU WANT TO BE PHYSICALLY FIT?

Important reasons for wanting to be physically fit	Enter your scores from p. 9	Circle if score is 12–10	Circle if score is 9–7	Circle if score is 6–4	Circle if score is 3
		THIS REASON IS			
HEART RATE AND RESPIRATORY RESERVE	_____	Most Important	Important	Somewhat Important	Least Important
STRESS AND TENSION RELIEF	_____	Most Important	Important	Somewhat Important	Least Important
ENERGY	_____	Most Important	Important	Somewhat Important	Least Important
MUSCLE TONE AND GENERAL CONDITIONING	_____	Most Important	Important	Somewhat Important	Least Important
FAT REDUCTION	_____	Most Important	Important	Somewhat Important	Least Important

You are ready to begin the next section, "Preparing for Fitness." The information you have learned about yourself from your "Profile Record" results will be useful to you when you actually choose your exercise program in Part 3, "Putting It All Together." But *before* you choose, read "Preparing for Fitness" and learn as much as you can about fitness, about establishing new patterns of activity, and about the general principles of exercise.

Most important, if you are interested in cardiorespiratory fitness, the concept of exercising in your target zone is essential. We will discuss the target zone in the second section of "Preparing for Fitness."

Part 2

Preparing for fitness

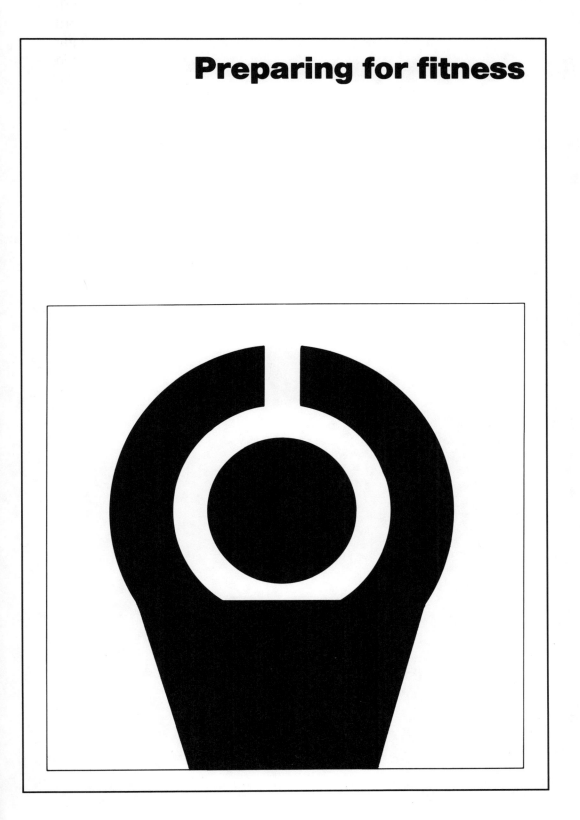

CHAPTER 3
Understanding physical fitness

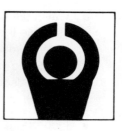

What is physical fitness? Physical fitness is difficult to define because it is related to your total health profile, not just your body's function. Fitness is related to your past medical history, family history, and your life-style and personal habits—smoking, eating, drinking, physical activity. (For detailed information about smoking behavior, nutrition, and safety and accident prevention, see other Health Action Plans.) Physical fitness can be measured by levels of respiratory capacity, heart rate, muscle tone, strength, stamina, and by proper weight. Put another way, physical fitness is what too many of us have lost. Typically when we are young we are physically active and participate in sports—hiking, bicycling, dancing. As we get older, we tend to become less active—riding instead of walking, dropping out of sports activities, sitting at desks, watching TV. The results are visible all around us—paunches, flabbiness, expanded waistlines, sagging posture, weak muscles, tension, and fatigue. There is something we can do about this. We can improve our way of living. We can eat more sensibly and moderately. We can eliminate harmful habits such as smoking. We can engage in suitable exercises and other physical activities that can help us develop and maintain physical fitness.

☐ Establishing new patterns of activity

The human body is a machine designed for action; it functions best only when the heart, blood vessels, lungs, muscles, skeleton, and nervous system receive adequate use. Before beginning a rigorous exercise program, think about—and act on—building new patterns of habitual movement. Start slowly, and gradually increase your activity level. For example:

- If you sit at a desk, get up each hour and walk briskly to the mail room or bathroom, down the hall, up some stairs—anything to get yourself moving.

- At lunchtime, take a brisk fifteen-minute walk before returning to work.

- Walk up and down stairs instead of taking an elevator; gradually increase the number of steps you climb before boarding elevators. When climbing stairs, inhale every other step and exhale in between. By regulating your breathing in this manner, you will not get winded as easily. Also when ascending stairs, do not lean forward and drag yourself up; stand straight and lift your entire body.

- Incorporate active recreation into your weekly schedule: bowling, swimming, dancing, cycling, jogging—plus walking. (Caution: if you enjoy competitive sports, do not leap from an inactive week into a weekend of vigorous tennis or basketball. It may dangerously tax your heart.)

- Limit your sedentary activities such as reading and watching television, or at best, be sure sedentary time is counteracted with active time.

- If you are a homemaker, do your housework vigorously. Turn on peppy music and work at an accelerated tempo.

- Set aside a specific amount of time each day to exercise. Try to make it the same time each day, such as before breakfast or after work. If you incorporate exercise into your routine, you will be less likely to get out of the habit.

☐ Caution: before beginning your fitness program

Before you start a fitness program, we recommend that you have a checkup performed by your physician, especially if you have not had a complete physical examination in the past year. It should include an examination of the heart and lungs. Your physician will decide if you need an electrocardiogram. It is generally advisable. It is especially important if you are over thirty-five and if you have ever been told by a physician that you have a heart problem or hypertension, or if others in your family have had such problems. If you wish to check your tolerance for exercise before you start your program, you should ask your physician about an exercise electrocardiogram or stress test.

In addition, check with your physician before exercising if you:

- Are a heavy smoker.

- Have been told by a physician that you have a thyroid disease.

- Have a family history of heart disease.

- Are more than 20 pounds overweight (see weight chart, page 132).

- Are over sixty and have never exercised.

■ Have had any chronic illness that may limit your ability to exercise, such as arthritis, rheumatism, gout, asthma, emphysema, or diabetes.

Remember, if you have a special physical problem, this may not mean that you cannot exercise. Special programs can be designed to suit your needs. Your physician can help you.

CHAPTER 4

Heart conditioning and your target zone

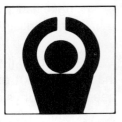

The key to increasing your fitness to its optimal level is the target-zone concept. A simple concept, it provides proof of improved heart and respiratory function. It especially allows you to judge whether you are exercising with the proper intensity to improve cardiac function, and whether you are doing it within safe limits. This valuable tool is important for endurance exercises like walking, jogging, skipping rope, dancing, bicycling, swimming, and jogging in place, which exercise the heart and lungs. The target-zone concept does not apply to exercises that strengthen muscles or improve flexibility, such as weight lifting or sit-ups.

Exercising stimulates the heart, the circulatory system, and the lungs. It causes more blood to flow to the heart from the veins; this increase in the supply of blood to the heart provides the resistance necessary to make the heart stronger—the heart needs this extra load (exercise beyond everyday activity) to condition it.

The target zone is the range within which you should exercise: the top of the range is 85 percent of your maximum heart rate; the bottom of the range is 70 percent of your maximum heart rate. Exercising within your target zone gives you the ability to increase your capacity for activity and actually have a reserve oxygen supply for extra energy.

An understanding of your heart or pulse rate (the terms are interchangeable) and your target zone will enable you to pace yourself as well as to measure your heart's progress. Your progress will be measured by a decrease in your heart rate: the slower your heart rate, the more efficient your cardiovascular system.

Any consistent exercise program—even walking—that provides additional work for the heart can succeed in lowering your resting pulse rate and improving the condition of your heart.

☐ How to find your resting pulse rate

There are several places on the body where your pulse or heart rate can be felt. Sit down for a minute. See if you can find your pulse on your wrist. Place the middle three fingers of one hand along the inner edge of the wrist, just below the base of the thumb. You may find it easier to count your pulse by holding your hand over your heart. A third method is to find the carotid artery located on either side of your neck under the angle of the jaw (the location is slightly different for each person).

Using a watch or clock with a second hand, feel the pulse or beat and count the beats for twenty seconds. Multiply this number by three

Beats counted for 20 seconds_____
Multiply this number by three_____
Equals your resting pulse rate_____

to get your heart or pulse rate per minute. This figure is your resting pulse rate.

☐ Tips about the resting pulse rate

Your resting pulse rate is an important indication of health. Men average 72 to 76 beats per minute, and women average 75 to 80 beats per minute. A general fitness program that includes endurance exercises will lower your resting pulse rate.

In general, the lower your resting pulse rate, the more efficient your heart and the healthier you are. If you are not in condition and have a pulse rate under 60, check with your doctor. You may have *bradycardia*—slow heart rate—due to a heart condition.

A high resting pulse rate means your body is working under a heavy load and your risk of coronary heart disease is increased.

☐ How to find your exercising pulse rate

Use a stopwatch or an ordinary watch or clock with a second hand. Jog in place for two minutes, raising your feet 4 to 5 inches from the floor.

Beats counted for six seconds_____
Add a zero to the figure above_____
Equals your exercising pulse rate_____

You should jog at the rate of 70–80 steps a minute; each time your left foot touches the floor counts as a step.

Immediately after exercising, feel your pulse and count the number of beats for six seconds. Because your heart rate drops off very quickly after exercising, a six-second reading is the most accurate. Add a zero to get your exercise pulse rate per minute.

☐ Finding your target zone

Your target zone is the minimum pulse rate and the maximum pulse rate within which your exercise program should take place. The minimum is where you *start* exercising; the maximum is what you *work toward.*

Your target zone is listed in the chart below. Locate your age range to find the minimum and maximum numbers that set the limits of your zone.

HEART RATE TARGET ZONE

Age range	Minimum-maximum
16–20	142–171
21–25	138–167
26–30	134–163
31–35	131–159
36–40	127–155
41–45	124–151
46–50	120–146
51–55	117–142
56–60	113–138
61–65	110–134
66–70	106–130
71–75	103–126

The above calculations are based on 220 minus age; 70 percent of 220 minus age gives you your minimum target zone, and 85 percent of 220 minus age gives you your maximum target zone.

These are estimates. If you find it too hard for you to exercise within the suggested target zone, perhaps it is too high for you. Your own individual target zone can be determined by an exercise tolerance test (stress test), if you wish to be more precise. This test must be administered by a physician.

□ The "perceived exertion method"

Of course, the best test for exertion is the response of your own body. You will quickly be able to tell if you are exerting too much or too little. Try to exercise at a level that you *perceive* to be moderate.

Taking note of your breathing can help you perceive the intensity of your exercise. If you breathe easily and can maintain a conversation, then the exercise is not too strenuous. If your breathing is interfering somewhat with the ease of talking but you can still maintain conversation, you are probably well within your target zone. But if your breathing is labored and painful, you are exercising too strenuously.

Use the estimated target zone on the chart to give you an idea of the approximate range of your heart activity. But take into account your perceptions of your body's response to exercise. If the estimated target zone is too high for you, don't be alarmed. Just exercise moderately, to the extent that seems comfortable for you.

☐ Progression

The ultimate goal of conditioning your heart is to *reduce your resting heart rate*. (Of course, if you are already in top-notch condition, the purpose of exercise is to *keep* you that way!) With regular, vigorous exercise, you can reduce your heart rate 5 to 10 beats per minute in a month's time.

In addition to reducing your resting heart rate, regular exercise will also reduce your exercising heart rate. As your heart becomes stronger, it will be more efficient. Therefore, it will take progressively more intense exercise for you to get your heart rate up into your target zone. In other words, to keep your heart at the same level over the course of training, you will have to exercise harder.

For example, at the beginning of training, fast walking may be sufficient to raise your heart rate into the target zone. After several months, you may find that you have to run for twenty or thirty minutes to reach the same heart rate.

Using the "perceived exertion method," you will notice that after several weeks you will feel no more strain doing vigorous exercise than you did doing mild exercise at the beginning of training. The same work load will feel easier; your breathing will be less strained. As time goes by, you can keep increasing your exercise load with no additional strain. As you progress and your cardiorespiratory system becomes conditioned, you will reach the stage where the oxygen you need to exercise in your target zone equals the oxygen that you use up without labored breathing. When this happens, some people experience a heightened sense of well-being during exercise.

☐ Caution: after starting your fitness program

After you have started your exercise program, you may find that you are doing too much too soon. The quickest way to discern whether or not you are overexerting is to check that your heartbeat remains within your target zone. Specifically, check your *recovery heart rate*. Five minutes after exercising, if your pulse rate is over 120, you are working too strenuously. After ten minutes, your pulse rate should be below 100.

The weather can affect how strenuously you should be exercising. If the weather is hot, and more so if it is humid, watch that you do not become overheated and dehydrated. Work out moderately, and drink lots of water.

Higher altitudes and friendly competition may also affect your heart rate. Without realizing it, you may be exercising too hard. Adjust your program if exercise is accompanied by:

- Prolonged fatigue.

- Breathlessness.

- A side stitch (muscle cramps in your abdomen or flanks).

- Muscle cramps.

- Aches and pains.

If you experience any of these signs, you are doing too much.

Stop your exercise program completely and see a physician if exercise is accompanied by:

- Chest pains or tightness in the chest.

- Great difficulty in breathing.

- Nausea.

- An abnormal heart rhythm.

- Dizziness, faintness, or light-headedness.

The results of your self-assessments together with an understanding of your target zone are the tools you need to put it all together. The next section outlines specifically which exercises are best to meet your goals, and it provides a chart to guide the planning of your program. Record-keeping suggestions and sample programs are discussed. After you read through these, you'll be ready to start your program. Be sure to refer to your ''Profile Record'' in Chapter 2 while devising your exercise program.

Part 3

Putting it all together

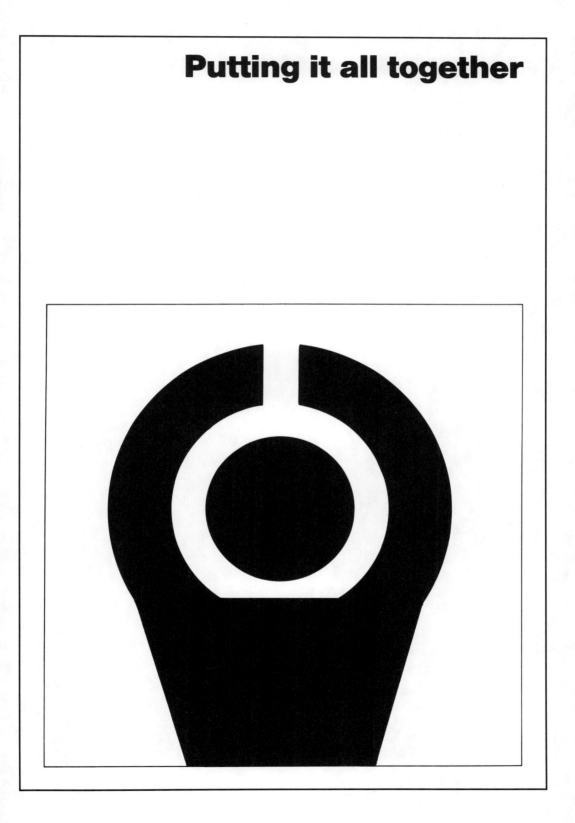

CHAPTER 5

General principles about exercising

To achieve maximum benefit from your exercise program, there are five basic principles to remember, and they apply to *all* exercise programs.

☐ Start exercising gradually

When you begin your exercise program, start at a light, easy level and *gradually* increase the intensity and amount of time spent doing a specific exercise. Try each exercise briefly the first time; allow yourself to become familiar with it. Don't overexert.

Take a close look at the reactions of your body. If you have been sedentary and immediately begin vigorous exercise, you will probably experience pain and soreness. Not only can this result in injury, but the pain can be so severe that you may be discouraged from continuing. Break yourself in gradually.

☐ Be specific about what you want exercise to do for you

Choose exercises that fit your goals. If you want to improve muscle strength and tone, you must make the specific muscles you want to strengthen work against more resistance than usual. If you want to improve flexibility, you must gently move your body to the limits of its range of motion. And if you want to improve cardiorespiratory function and endurance, engage the large muscles of the body for several minutes at a time. Total fitness will involve all of these.

☐ Consider intensity and duration

The intensity with which you exercise together with the length of time you exercise constitute the *extra-load principle.* The extra-load principle means simply that you must expose your body to more exercise than it is normally accustomed to in order to improve its fitness. The greater the intensity of the activity and the longer it is carried on, the greater the stimulation to the muscles and the cardiovascular system.

Remember, however, that if the extra load is too great, you may experience pain and soreness that can be detrimental. Also, exercises should be tempered so that your pulse remains within your heart rate target zone (see page 20).

☐ Include a warm-up phase and a cool-down phase

Always limber up your muscles and gently stimulate your blood circulation before starting your vigorous activity. Warming up protects your muscles and joints from sudden strain and injury.

Never stop cold after exercising vigorously. A sudden stop can cause blood to pool in your extremities and can make you dizzy or faint. Cool down with gentle exercises or slower movement.

☐ Exercise regularly

Exercise must be done frequently and habitually for a minimum of three days per week to ensure that gains are maintained. Chapter 7, "A Guide to Planning Your Fitness Program," explains which kinds of exercise will help you meet your goals (from Part 1, "Self-Assessment"). But remember, a good exercise program can help you achieve more than one goal. All exercise expends calories. A program to strengthen the heart will result in extra energy; a muscle-conditioning program will help you to relax; even moderate exercises will strengthen your muscles and help trim your figure. Exercises that result in cardiovascular fitness, however, rely upon vigorous beating of the heart for a sustained period of time—twenty to thirty minutes— at least three times per week. Sports activities such as swimming, tennis, racketball, bicycling, jogging, and exercises such as jogging in place or skipping rope can help achieve cardiovascular fitness.

CHAPTER 6

The basic health action plan for physical fitness

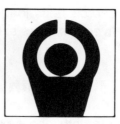

Now that you know the general principles for any exercise regimen, you can begin to devise your individual Health Action Plan for physical fitness. Any exercise regimen that follows the Health Action Plan guidelines will have these two qualities:

- By incorporating exercises to fulfill each of the categories of fitness, you will have a regimen for *total* fitness.

- Because you are able to choose from a wide variety of exercises, your program will be suited to your *personal needs and desires.*

The Health Action Plan exercises, which are described in detail in Part 4, are organized under six basic categories: warm-up, endurance, strength, flexibility, cool-down, and relaxation. With each group of exercises is an explanation of how to do each exercise and how to incorporate them into your program.

☐ Warm-up exercises

The warm-up phase of your program should last five minutes. The warm-up is designed to increase the circulation of blood to the muscles, to raise body temperature, and to increase the heart rate gradually until it reaches the target zone (see page 20.)

To warm up, you can do the suggested warm-up exercises, work at your endurance exercise at a slower, easier pace, or combine a few strength and flexibility exercises with a few minutes of your slow-paced endurance exercise. No matter which method you choose, be sure to warm up for the *full five minutes.*

☐ Endurance exercises

The endurance phase is central to any exercise program. The goal of any endurance exercise is to increase cardiorespiratory stamina, the most important part of physical fitness. Endurance exercises include such vigorous exercises as jogging, bicycling, and swimming. You should spend at least *twenty minutes* exercising within your target zone.

☐ Strength and flexibility exercises

Strength and flexibility exercises should be included in any total fitness program to assure that every muscle and joint will receive at least some attention. These exercises may be the chief component of your self-designed program or they may be incorporated into the cool-down phase of your activities.

Strength exercises are designed to improve overall muscle strength and tone, and to protect the body from injury; flexibility exercises are designed to limber muscles and joints. You might also select a particular strength or flexibility exercise to work on a specific group of muscles, such as those in the legs or torso, that may require special attention. Study your "Profile Record," pages 10–11, to see which areas might need work, and select your exercises accordingly.

Remember, in any program spend at least five minutes concentrating on strength and flexibility, both to condition your body and to cool down after doing your endurance exercise. We suggest that you spend approximately two minutes on strength and three minutes on flexibility, always ending with a flexibility exercise.

☐ Cool-down

The cool-down phase is as important as the warm-up phase. Spend *five minutes* keeping up activity but not with the same intensity. Strength and flexibility exercises, done without strain, can be incorporated into the cool-down.

Cooling down is a transition back to your baseline state of physical activity. It is a time of physiologic readjustment. You should never stop suddenly after exercising vigorously, because a sudden stop can make you feel dizzy or faint. Never sit down or lie down after a vigorous workout; instead, spend about five minutes exercising at a slower pace to allow your body to cool down and your pulse rate to return to normal.

☐ Relaxation

We strongly suggest that after you cool down you finish your exercise routine with a few minutes of *complete relaxation*. You may do this by just reclining comfortably and dwelling on pleasant thoughts or listening to music, or you may wish to do the relaxation exercise suggested on page 76. In addition, in Part 6, we suggest several programs for relaxation and relief of tension, and you may wish to include one or more of these, such as meditation or massage, in your regular exercise regimen.

The relaxation phase should serve to reinforce the benefits of the entire workout. Think over what you have achieved in the last twenty or thirty minutes. That should make you feel good and give you a sense of satisfaction. It should also refresh your mind for whatever you do next, whether it is going to sleep or going to work.

☐ Other tips

Plan, in general, to work out at least three times per week. Exercising every other day seems to be an effective way to exercise regularly because it allows time between sessions for the body to recover from the previous workout and thus slowly adapt to a higher level. As you become better conditioned, you can exercise more often.

We emphasize the importance of building up gradually to allow the muscles to adapt to the new stresses. It is common for people unaccustomed to exercise to develop aches and pains when starting an exercise program. After a week or two, you may want to increase the number of workouts per week or the amount of time per workout, but don't try too much too soon. The best guide is the way you feel.

☐ Special programs

In addition to "The Basic Health Action Plan for Physical Fitness," we have included a few special programs to suit specific needs.

The moderate exercise programs in Chapter 15 are designed for elderly people or for those who for health or other reasons might require a less vigorous regimen. One program features a variety of exercises; the second is a detailed walking routine.

Lower-back pain is a problem that affects thousands of people. If you have back-pain problems due to muscle weakness, Chapter 18, "Lower-Back Pain Prevention and Relief Program," should help you deal with your problem.

Finally, because relaxing effectively is as important as exercising effectively, we have included several programs for relaxation and relief of tension. These are:

- Relaxation techniques
- Isometrics
- Yoga-type exercises
- Meditation
- Massage

Consider including one of these in the relaxation phase of your basic program. For example, meditation and massage can easily be included in a basic program. Also, on alternate days (days you are not doing your complete program), you may want to do isometrics or yoga-type exercises. Think, too, about incorporating some of the "Selected Relaxation Techniques" into your everyday life (see page 102).

CHAPTER 7

A guide to planning your fitness program

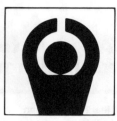

Using "The Basic Health Action Plan for Physical Fitness" and taking into account your personal goals identified on the "Profile Record," choose exercises for each of the program phases: warm-up, endurance, strength and flexibility, cool-down, and relaxation. Select exercises that you enjoy, and, to avoid boredom, make substitutions occasionally. Make it a social experience: exercise with one or more friends!

Set your own pace. For the most part, the time frames suggested are not absolute—except for the endurance phase, which requires that you exercise within your target zone for a full twenty minutes. However, if you wish to warm up longer, or to concentrate for a greater length of time on strength and flexibility, feel free to do so. Remember not to strain in the beginning. Read the text section preceding each of the groups of exercises in Part 4 carefully, and take special note of the tips that are offered.

A guide to planning your fitness program

Health action plan exercises	Goals	Guidelines to choosing exercises
EXERCISES FOR WARMING UP pp. 42–46	■ To prepare the body for exercise. ■ To increase circulation to the muscles. ■ To gradually increase heart rate.	No matter which program you follow, include *5 minutes* of warm-up.
EXERCISES FOR ENDURANCE pp. 47–59	■ To strengthen the heart. ■ To improve respiratory function. ■ To trim the figure and improve muscle tone.	See "Self-Assessment 3" on "Profile Record." If you scored high (7–12) in "Heart Rate and Respiratory," "Energy," or "Fat Reduction," endurance exercises are essential to meet your goal(s). Do *20 minutes* of endurance exercises. If you scored high (23 or over) on your composite score in "Self-Assessment 3," you are prepared to start at a vigorous level. If you scored low, work up gradually. Endurance exercises can be strenuous; stay within your target zone. If you have a low composite score, start exercising at your minimum target zone level.
EXERCISES FOR STRENGTH pp. 60–65	■ To improve muscle strength specifically or overall. ■ To improve muscle tone. ■ To protect the body from injury, and prevent the development of aches and pains.	See "Self-Assessment 3" on "Profile Record." If you scored high (7–12) in "Muscle Tone and General Conditioning," concentrate on exercises for strength.
EXERCISES FOR FLEXIBILITY pp. 66–75	■ To improve flexibility of muscles and joints. ■ To improve agility and coordination.	See "Self-Assessment 3" on "Profile Record." If you scored high (7–12) in "Muscle Tone and General Conditioning" or "Stress and Tension Relief," concentrate on exercises for flexibility.

Health action plan exercises	Goals	Guidelines to choosing exercises
EXERCISES FOR COOLING DOWN p. 76	■ To prepare your body for relaxation. ■ To decrease heart rate, gradually.	Alternate strength and flexibility exercises. End with a flexibility exercise. Cool down for a total of *5 minutes* when using strength and flexibility exercises as part of a general fitness program, after endurance exercises.
EXERCISES FOR RELAXATION pp. 76–77	■ To eliminate tension from your body. ■ To allow time to contemplate the feeling of well-being and benefit after exercising. ■ To lower your pulse rate to your resting pulse rate.	No matter which program you follow, include a *few minutes* of relaxation.

	Goals	Guidelines to choosing exercises
MODERATE FITNESS PROGRAMS p. 79–98	■ To improve muscle tone, circulation, and joint flexibility. ■ To improve cardiovascular fitness and energy.	If you are over 60 and/or scored low (below 14) on your composite score in "Self-Assessment 2," begin exercising with one of the moderate programs.

Special programs	Goals	Guidelines to choosing special programs
PROGRAMS FOR RELAXATION AND RELIEF OF TENSION pp. 101–17	■ To eliminate fatigue and increase energy. ■ To relieve stress.	See "Self-Assessment 3" on "Profile Record." If you scored high (7–12) in "Stress and Tension Relief" or "Energy," the relaxation programs are for you. Choose from those provided.
LOWER-BACK PAIN PREVENTION AND RELIEF PROGRAM pp. 118–26	■ To strengthen lower-back and abdominal muscles. ■ To eliminate lower-back pain. ■ To prevent back problems. ■ To improve posture.	If you have back pain that has no organic cause, or you wish to improve your posture, incorporate this program into your routine. This program will help strengthen your back and abdominal muscles.

☐ Sample programs

Here are three sample programs to help guide you in planning your own exercise regimen. Keep in mind your ultimate goals as you plan your program. Check the "Profile Record" and note areas where you are weak or would like to be stronger. With this information in mind, you may choose to emphasize one area more than another. For example, you may wish to strengthen muscles. In this case, add more strength exercises to your basic program. Don't forget that a program should be pleasurable! Choose exercises you know you will enjoy.

The total exercise time for each sample program is thirty-five minutes. Time can be varied according to your level of fitness. You may start out with shorter exercise periods and work up, or spend more time warming up and less time with endurance.

If followed regularly three times per week, any one of these sample programs will work well as a constructive fitness program.

The total time of each program is 35 minutes. This can be varied according to your level of fitness. You may start out with shorter time frames and build up to these. These time frames are good for a maintenance program, if done three times a week.

SAMPLE PROGRAM 1

Phase	Exercise	Time
Warm-up	Walking	5 minutes
Endurance	Jogging	20 minutes
Cool-down: Strength	Body twists Half-knee bends	2 minutes
Flexibility	Head rotation Shoulder-level arm swings Alternating leg bends	3 minutes
Relaxation	Meditation	5 minutes
		TOTAL TIME 35 minutes

SAMPLE PROGRAM 2

Phase	Exercise	Time
Warm-up	Head rotation Up and down stretch Side twist	3 minutes
	Skipping rope (slowly)	2 minutes
Endurance	Skipping rope	20 minutes
Cool-down: Strength	Abdominal curl Graduated pushups	2 minutes
Flexibility	Body twists Shoulder-level arm swings Toe touching	3 minutes
Relaxation	Deep breathing	5 minutes
		TOTAL TIME 35 minutes

SAMPLE PROGRAM 3

Phase	Exercise	Time
Warm-up	Alternating leg bends Head rotation Side bends	5 minutes
Endurance	Jogging in place Jumping jacks Side hops	20 minutes
Cool-down: Strength	Body twists Weight raiser Side leg raise (on hands and knees)	3 minutes
Flexibility	Forward and backward bend Shoulder-level arm swings	2 minutes
Relaxation	Yoga exercises	5 minutes
		TOTAL TIME 35 minutes

□ Record keeping

It is very important that you keep a record as you do your exercises. By creating a chart similar to the one on the opposite page, you can maintain an ongoing record of precisely what you have accomplished. We also suggest that you keep notes regarding how you feel both mentally and physically—and you can be sure that as you advance in your program, you will feel better both mentally and physically!

After each exercise session, carefully fill in your chart. It is especially important to check your resting pulse rate each week and compare it with the previous week's figure. In the first two weeks of exercise, it is also important to record your exercising pulse rate and your recovery rates. If they fall outside the desired zones, adjust your program accordingly.

Exercise record
(sample)

	DAY 1	DAY 2	DAY 3
Resting pulse rate	75	85	80
WARM-UP			
Exercise	Walking	Head rotation, up + down stretch, side twist, skip rope slowly	Head rotation, side bends, leg bends
Time	5 minutes	5 minutes	5 minutes
Exercising pulse rate	100	110	105
STIMULUS PERIOD (endurance exercise)			
Exercise	Jogging	Skipping rope	Jogging in place, side hops, jumping jacks
Time	20 minutes	20 minutes	20 minutes
Exercise pulse rate	135	148	137
STRENGTH			
Exercise	Body twists + half-knee bends	Abdominal curl + graduated pushups	Side leg raise, body twist, weight raiser
Time	2 minutes	2 minutes	3 minutes
FLEXIBILITY			
Exercise	Head rotation, shoulder-level arm swings, leg bends	Body twists, toe touching, arm swings	arm swing, forward + backward bends
Time	3 minutes	3 minutes	2 minutes
RELAXATION			
Exercise	Meditation	Deep breathing	Yoga exercises
Time	5 minutes	5 minutes	5 minutes
Total time	35 minutes	35 minutes	35 minutes
Recovery rate (pulse rate) After 5 minutes	95	98	100
After 10 minutes	85	92	94
Notes	Feel tired. Glad I started a regular program. Hope this keeps weight down.	Skipping rope was hard, but relaxation helps me recover from aches and pains. Feels good.	Feels good to exercise after a long day at office. Refreshed + ready for a good evening.

Health action plan exercises

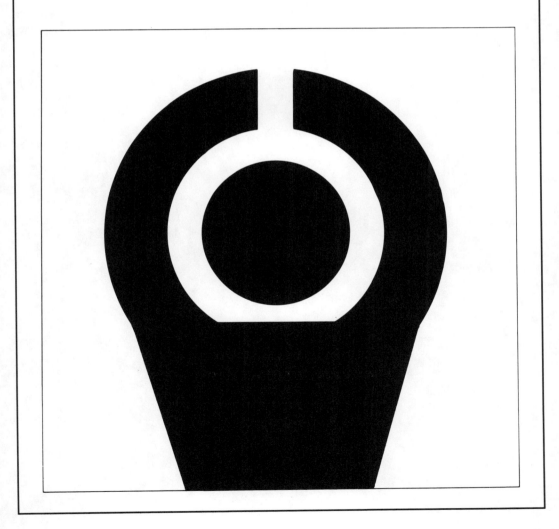

CHAPTER 8
Introduction

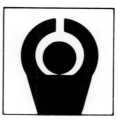

Part 4 discusses and illustrates the different categories of exercises: warm-up, endurance, strength, flexibility, and relaxation. By choosing from these categories and using the time frames provided in the sample programs (pages 34–35) as well as the "Guide to Planning Your Fitness Program" (pages 32–33), you can create a personalized exercise program. Depending on your goals, you may wish to increase the time allocated for strength or flexibility exercises.

Review each exercise and note which ones appeal most to you. Using a sheet of paper, leave spaces between the categories, and jot down the warm-up, endurance, strength, flexibility, and relaxation exercises that you would enjoy doing. Some will seem more worth doing and more suitable for your goals. Check off exercises under strength and flexibility that you wish to do for your cool-down.

Once you have a list of your preferred and most appropriate exercises, you have only to follow the sample record-keeping sheet and to use the suggested time frames, and you're on your way toward fitness.

Remember, although the instructions for each exercise suggest the number of repetitions to be done, these are somewhat arbitrary and you can vary them according to your own needs.

CHAPTER 9
Warm-up exercises

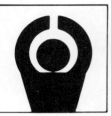

A warming-up phase is an absolute necessity for any fitness program. In order to avoid strain and injury, the body must be brought from a state of rest to a state of work before beginning vigorous exercise. Specifically, warm-up exercises increase circulation to the muscles, increase body temperature, and raise the heart rate gradually until it reaches its target zone (see page 20).

A warm-up routine should last a minimum of five minutes to be sure the body is prepared. Warm-up exercises should always be done *slowly*. Do not stretch your muscles to the limit of your range of motion. Move them easily and gradually.

You can incorporate the warming-up phase into your fitness program in any one of three ways:

1 You can use any of the flexibility exercises in Chapter 12, but for warming up, do these exercises at a slow pace. Do not stretch your muscles to the extreme; work up gently.

2 You can perform your selected endurance exercise for the first five minutes at a slower, easier pace. For example, jog slowly, swim one or two laps at a gentle pace, or bicycle for one mile at an easy rate.

3 You can combine a few of the flexibility exercises with a slowed-down version of your endurance exercise. For example, you may wish to do three minutes of flexibility exercises and then slowly begin your endurance exercise for two minutes.

No matter which method you choose, be sure to exercise at a slow rate for at least five minutes before beginning your endurance exercise. Move slowly, stretch gently, and gradually get your body warm, limber, and ready for more vigorous activity.

Alternating leg bends

Purpose
To stretch muscles of legs, hips, waist, buttocks, and lower back.

Starting position
Place feet far apart with legs straight. Place hands on knees and lean forward from the waist.

Action
1 Bend right knee.

2 Return to starting position.

3 Bend left knee.

4 Return to starting position.

5 Repeat steps 1 through 4 four times.

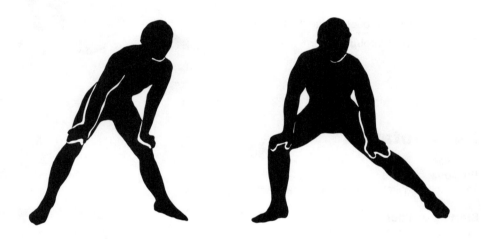

Sitting single-leg raise

Purpose
To stretch muscles of your abdomen, waist, and thighs.

Starting position
Sit on the floor with knees bent and feet flat on the floor. Place your hands on the floor behind you for support. Keep moving your hands farther back until you find a position that is comfortable for you. Keep arms straight and elbows locked.

Action
1 Extend your right leg slowly upward until it is straight.

2 Point your toes as you extend your leg.

3 Lower your right leg smoothly to the starting position.

4 Repeat steps 1 through 3 with the left leg.

5 Repeat steps 1 through 4 four times.

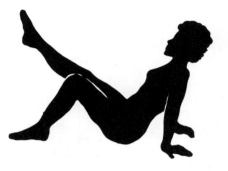

Head rotation

Purpose
To stretch and limber neck and upper back.

Starting position
Stand erect but relaxed, with feet shoulder-width apart and arms behind your back. Look straight ahead.

Action
1 Let head fall forward and then far to the right in one smooth motion until you can look at the floor behind your right shoulder. Reverse the motion and return to the starting position.

2 Let your head fall forward and to the left in one smooth motion until you can look at the floor behind your left shoulder. Reverse the motion and return to the starting position.

3 Repeat 1 and 2, alternating the motion from right to left.

4 Repeat steps 1 through 3 four times.

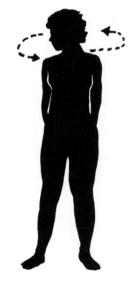

Up and down stretch

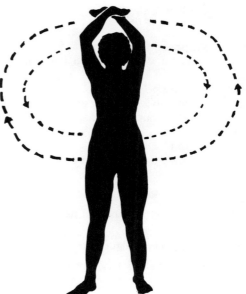

Purpose
To stretch muscles of arms, shoulders, chest, and upper back.

Starting position
Stand erect with feet shoulder-width apart and arms hanging loosely at your sides.

Action
1 Raise and stretch arms over your head until wrists touch.

2 Stretch arms in a circle downward until wrists touch in front of your abdomen.

3 Repeat steps 1 and 2 ten to twelve times.

Shoulder-level arm swings

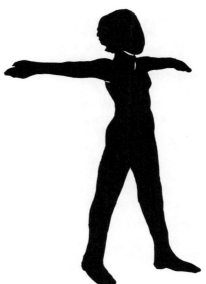

Purpose
To limber shoulders and upper arms.

Starting position
Stand erect with feet shoulder-width apart. Thrust chest out and stretch arms out sideways at shoulder level with palms up.

Action
1 With fingers closed into a fist, swing arms forward, keeping arms straight.

2 As arms come together, open fists and clap your hands gently in front of you.

3 Swing arms slowly back to starting position with chest thrust out and fingers wide open.

4 Repeat steps 1 through 3 ten to twelve times.

Side twist

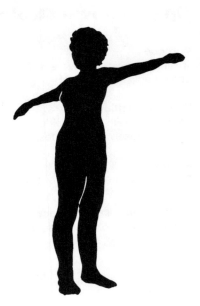

Purpose
To limber waist, abdomen, and sides.

Starting position
Stand with feet comfortably apart and arms extended out to the sides, palms down.

Action
1 Slowly twist the upper part of your body to your left.
2 Return to starting position.
3 Slowly twist the upper part of your body to your right.
4 Return to starting position.
5 Repeat steps 1 through 4 four times.

Side bends (one arm raised)

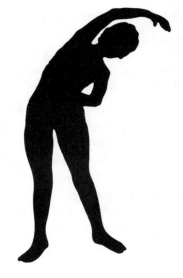

Purpose
To stretch and limber waist, back muscles, vertebrae, and sacroiliac joints.

Starting position
Stand erect with feet slightly wider than shoulder-width apart. Place right arm behind your back and raise your left arm straight above your head.

Action
1 With chest thrust forward, shoulders back, and abdomen tucked in, bend your body to the right until you feel a slight pull at your waist. Hold the position for 4 seconds.
2 Repeat step 1 four times.
3 Reverse position of arms and repeat steps 1 and 2 to the left side.

> **Remember, warm-up exercises are a preliminary step to the endurance exercises that follow.**

CHAPTER 10

Endurance exercises

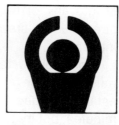

Endurance exercises are those that you must perform for twenty minutes or more to promote cardiovascular fitness. Frequently, endurance exercises are activities of locomotion involving large muscle groups in which the entire body is moved, such as walking, running, swimming, cycling, dancing, or skipping rope.

Endurance is dependent upon your body's ability to take in oxygen, transport it to the working muscles, and utilize it to liberate the energy needed to do the vigorous exercise. Endurance depends on the sound functioning of the lungs, heart, and circulatory system. At the same time, endurance exercises can improve the functioning of these organs as well as build the muscles that are performing the work.

Increasing the cardiac capacity to work is perhaps the most important aspect of the endurance part of the exercise program. Exercising within your heart rate target zone is imperative. Reread Chapter 4, "Heart Conditioning and Your Target Zone," and take care throughout your exercise training program that you increase your exercise sufficiently so that the heart muscle is steadily strengthened.

The endurance phase of your fitness program is the pivotal part of training. Endurance exercises should be performed for a minimum of ten minutes, and twenty to thirty minutes is really better. (After thirty minutes of strenuous exercise, more time gives proportionately less benefit.) Choose an exercise that you enjoy and that is easily accessible to you.

☐ Walking

Walking is the simplest and most convenient endurance exercise. Anyone can include a regular schedule of walking in his or her everyday life, and it is a particularly convenient exercise for those who are overweight, out of shape, middle-aged, elderly, or have been extremely inactive. If you fit into any of these categories, a more vigorous exercise might be too strenuous at first and walking is a good way to begin to get the body into shape.

For walking to be effective, it must be approached purposefully and must be done at a brisk pace every day. Do not stroll or saunter, but establish a pace of 3 to 4 miles per hour. At first, walk for about twenty minutes, but try to quickly work up to longer periods.

Of course, the pace and distance you walk are determined by your capacity. Vigorous walking for twenty minutes with warm-up and cool-down periods of five minutes each is a good way to start. As with each endurance exercise, keep the heart rate in the target zone for the entire walk.

As you get into better shape, you may want to slowly work up to a jogging program.

Walking regularly and vigorously over progressively longer periods of time trims the body and strengthens and tones the muscles, especially the leg muscles. Walking keeps the joints flexible and improves circulation, digestion, and sleep. In addition, it can help you lose weight.

Walking is a versatile exercise, either as the primary endurance exercise in an overall fitness program or as a warm-up exercise for a jogging, rope skipping, or dancing program (or virtually any other endurance exercise program). It can also be used as an ''auxiliary exercise''—to be done on those days when doing the regular exercise is impossible.

For additional information about walking as exercise, see Chapter 16, ''A Walking Program.''

☐ Jogging

Jogging is steady, slow running; in a full program it can be interspersed with periods of walking. It is one of the best endurance exercises because it strengthens the heart, lungs, and circulatory system by gradually expanding their capacity to handle stress. Jogging also helps you look better. It redistributes your weight (and can help you lose weight, if that is your goal), trims the waist, and flattens the abdomen. It also firms muscles, particularly in the legs.

Jogging can be enjoyed by almost anyone because a program can be modified to suit any physical condition. You can even begin a jogging program with the walking program, slowly working up to a faster pace.

A JOGGING PROGRAM

To prevent pain, stiffness, cramps, or other injury, it is wise to spend a few *extra* minutes warming up before jogging. Instead of the standard five, warm up for six or seven minutes, selecting exercises to limber the upper body, neck, and, of course, the legs. You also might try doing warm-up exercises for five minutes, walking for two minutes, and then jogging.

At the beginning of your jogging program, jog only two or three times a week to begin to get your body into condition. On alternate days, substitute other endurance exercises such as walking, bicycling, or swimming to keep muscles limber.

As you are conditioning yourself for jogging, alternate brisk walking with actual jogging. Set 1 mile as your limit at first. When you begin you may have to jog for one minute and then walk for one minute. Each day try to jog longer than the day before and walk less, until you can jog for the entire mile. As you improve, you will be able to jog farther and faster. You will have to keep lengthening your course in order to get a full twenty minutes of exercise.

Undoubtedly you will walk more than you will jog at first. But you should quickly improve. If you become breathless, slow down. If you find you need an extra day's rest, take it. If you experience extreme breathlessness, pain in the chest, nausea, or pounding in the head while jogging, stop immediately. These are signs that you have gone *beyond* the limits of your present tolerance. Build your tolerance by doing one of the less strenuous endurance exercises, and then go back to jogging.

After your exercise session, finish with about five minutes of stretching, strengthening, and flexibility exercises. Then relax completely.

GUIDELINES FOR JOGGING

- Always wear good, well-cushioned jogging shoes. These are essential. Buy the best pair you can afford. Jogging with sneakers or gym shoes can lead to foot, shin, knee, or back injury. The shoes should have a slight lift in the heel. Be sure they fit perfectly.

- Wear loose, comfortable clothing. Sweat socks are particularly important because they keep feet dry and supple. A jogging bra may be comfortable for some women. In cold weather, wear several layers of lightweight sweaters, a windbreaker, and a wool cap. (You will perspire even in winter; a cap helps prevent colds.) In hot and humid weather, jog during the coolest part of the day. Drink plenty of water.

- Never wear rubberized or plastic clothing. These can produce dehydration and heat exhaustion.

- When jogging, make sure you step down on your entire foot so your weight is distributed evenly, not just on your toes or the balls of your feet. Hold your head erect. Try to relax all your muscles and breathe regularly through your nose and mouth. You should not be breathless; you should be able to carry on a conversation while jogging. Learn to pace yourself. Do not try to do more than your body is ready to handle.

- To make sure that shin muscles stay limber and strong, try these two exercises. First, flex your feet as though you are trying to touch your shin with your toes. Repeat five flexes with one leg, five with the other. Second, while sitting in a chair, extend your legs forward until they are straight.

- Make sure the warm-up and cool-down phases of your program last at least five minutes each. The actual jogging time should be fifteen to twenty minutes, during which your heart functions in the target zone.

- Your jogging surface should not be hard. Try to jog only on resilient surfaces such as dirt or grass. Concrete and asphalt are too hard and put added stress on your legs and feet. (Proper jogging shoes can compensate for this to some extent.) Also, avoid uneven surfaces such as sandy beaches. Watch out for roots, stumps, curbs, and other obstacles—they can trip you.

- A highly effective warm-up for stretching the muscles in the back of the lower leg and the Achilles tendon is to stand about 2 feet from a wall, tree, or lamppost, place both hands flat on its surface at shoulder height, and lean forward at about a 45-degree angle. Keep both heels flat on the ground. Lean into the wall with your knees and hips straight until you feel a pull behind the knee or in the lower leg. Increase the tension gradually. A warm-up for stretching the hamstring muscle, which is behind the thigh, is to stand, extend one leg forward, and rest it on a counter, chair, or railing about 3 feet high. While keeping the other leg straight, attempt to touch the toes of the extended leg with both hands. It may take several weeks to be able to do this. Alternate legs for several minutes.

☐ Swimming

Swimming is an excellent all-around endurance exercise. It uses virtually all the muscles in the body without placing too much strain on any part. Many people, including the elderly and very sedentary, enjoy exercising in water and find it easier. While exercising in water actually requires more energy, it *seems* to require less effort than exercising on land. A swimming exercise program, like any other, should be structured so that you exercise different muscle groups, exercise within your target zone, and of course, warm up and cool down.

The stroke that provides the best cardiovascular workout is the Australian crawl—propelling yourself on your abdomen, arm over arm, head turning rhythmically in and out of the water. The breaststroke and the sidestroke are less taxing. The backstroke employs little-used muscle groups and requires more effort, but it is an enjoyable variation. It is good to vary your strokes (especially those employing your arm muscles) to avoid fatigue, and using a variety of strokes enhances enjoyment and reduces boredom.

A SWIMMING PROGRAM

It is easier to carry out a swimming program in a pool than in a lake or ocean. If you do swim in natural bodies of water, be sure to swim parallel to the shore. Don't swim alone.

Start with five minutes of warm-up exercises. You can select a few activities from the flexibility exercises in Chapter 12 or warm up by swimming very slowly for the first few minutes.

After warming up, swim vigorously for twenty minutes, not necessarily continuously; rest when you have to. Gradually work up to your target zone. Whatever stroke you choose you will be strengthening muscles, limbering joints, and exercising your heart. Some find it helpful to swim one or more laps, get out, walk the length of the pool, and then begin again. Swimming laps in a pool is an important but not the only water exercise. A useful supplementary or alternative program consists of exercises in the water. Most of these can also be done by nonswimmers in shallow water.

FLUTTER KICK

Lying flat on your abdomen, hold on to the side of the pool, to a friend, or to a kickboard. Point your toes and kick your legs, flutter style. Keep your ankles flexible and your knees loose, but your legs straight.

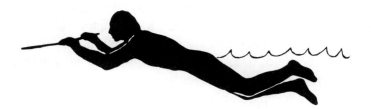

BOB AND SQUAT

Stand in a vertical position in water up to your shoulders. With hands over your head, bend your knees until you are in a squatting position entirely underwater, then rapidly jump up out of the water. Inhale at the peak of your rise out of the water. You're actually jumping up and down in the water from a squat position to an extended vertical position.

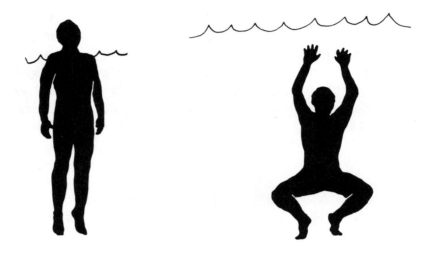

LEG RAISE

Alternately raise your legs while lying on your back in the water and paddling with your arms to keep yourself afloat. Bring left knee to chest, then straighten the left leg so that it is perpendicular to the water's surface. Return to lying position. Alternate with your right leg. If this is done in shallow water, your arms can be supporting you by resting on the bottom of the pool. This exercise should be attempted only by experienced swimmers.

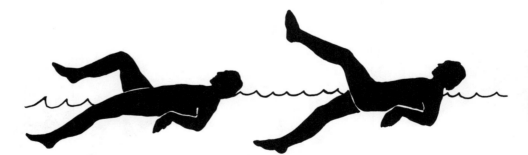

DOG PADDLE

Dog paddling can be an excellent exercise. Most people learn to swim by discovering the dog paddle. It's almost an instinctive motion that doesn't need much explanation. Paddling is akin to pedaling a bicycle, but your arms "pedal" or paddle also. Both arms remain underwater all the time, your elbows stay close to the body, not out to the side, and the arms paddle forward underwater. The arm action need not be vigorous to keep you afloat and it may be varied. Another arm action is to turn your palms outward in front of your chest and then push the water away from your body. Then turn your palms inward and bring your hands together. Keep your hands fairly straight as you repeat these movements. This action of pushing water with the palms is called "sculling" and is a great aid in maintaining buoyancy. Paddle or scull and kick at the same time; let your knees bend more than you normally would. Practice in shallow water and then go to somewhat deeper water and paddle.

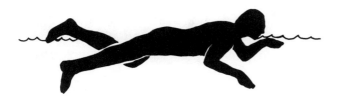

The above four exercises should be done for one to three minutes each, depending on individual preferences. Repeating the cycle twice will take about twenty minutes.

You may wish to combine swimming and some water exercises for the twenty minutes of your endurance phase. Make sure you cool down by swimming slowly for about five minutes, or follow the cool-down routine suggested previously: two minutes of strength exercises and three minutes of flexibility exercises.

Start by swimming three times per week on nonconsecutive days. This is sufficient, but you may wish to progress to five times a week. As you progress, you will have to increase the distance you swim within the twenty-minute endurance period to keep your heart rate in its proper target zone. You may also wish to increase the amount of time you swim, or the duration of your water exercising.

For those who have access to a pool, swimming is a sport that should be seriously considered for an excellent, enjoyable, all-around fitness program.

☐ Skipping rope

Skipping rope is an excellent method for developing cardiopulmonary fitness. The only equipment you need is the rope itself. You may need a bit of practice before you achieve the rhythm and coordination necessary to do continuous jumping, but basically it is a simple sport.

A SKIPPING-ROPE PROGRAM

Before jumping, warm up for five minutes with a few exercises selected from among those in the warm-up phase (see Chapter 9). Include a minute of moderate rope jumping as part of your warming-up session.

Jump rope for fifteen minutes, taking breaks if you have to. Try to work out five times a week, or a minimum of three times per week on non-consecutive days. The fifteen-minute time limit can be altered to suit your age and physical condition. Skipping rope raises the heart level rapidly, so watch your heart-rate target-zone limit.

Start jumping at a modest level and do not overexert yourself. If you become breathless, stop for a bit. Do not, however, stand still or sit down. Walk around until you feel ready to jump again. Alternate jumping with walking.

A modest program might be to skip 20 steps, then walk, then skip another 20 steps until the fifteen minutes is up. Gradually increase the skips until the entire session is rope skipping. If 20 skips is too easy, increase the number. Find a pace that suits you.

After your rope-skipping routine, cool down for five minutes.

GUIDELINES FOR SKIPPING ROPE

- Do not skip barefooted; this is hard on feet and legs. Wear absorbent flat-heeled shoes such as sneakers.

- Skip as lightly as possible, landing on the balls of your feet.

- Use your wrists, not your arms, to turn the rope. The wrist action keeps you from tiring too quickly.

- Always stop before the point of breathlessness. Count out loud while skipping, and check periodically to see that your heart is functioning within your target zone.

- Make a jump rope from # 10 sash cord or clothesline rope purchased from a hardware store. To determine the right length for you, stand on the rope with your feet together and lift the rope so that it comes to just beneath your armpits. Cut the rope to this length and knot the ends. Also, professional ropes can be purchased from sporting goods stores.

- Once you achieve your fitness level, you can maintain it by engaging in this exercise three times a week on nonconsecutive days.

☐ Dancing

Dancing can be an excellent conditioning activity if it is done regularly, at least three times a week on alternate days. Dancing must be done intensively enough so that your heart rate remains within your target zone for at least twenty minutes. This type of dancing—sometimes called "aerobic dancing"—not only improves your circulatory and respiratory systems, but also tones muscles and improves posture, coordination, balance, and agility.

You do not have to be an accomplished dancer to participate in a dance program, nor do you have to use conventional dance steps. All you have to do is keep your body moving rhythmically at a pace that is right for you. Extend your arms and legs, bend and stretch your torso, move from side to side, lift your feet, raise your head. Do all of these movements to music. You will improve muscle tone, increase your strength and flexibility, and improve your coordination. Dance to music and rhythms that you like, using any steps or patterns. The only requirement is to make sure you are exercising strenuously enough so that your heart rate is in the required target zone and remains there for fifteen or twenty minutes.

A DANCE PROGRAM

Precede your dancing with a warm-up period. Select exercises from the warm-up exercises in Chapter 9. You might try exercising to music to get you in the mood to dance.

Because of the wide variety of tempos and movements, it is difficult to prescribe a set pattern of dance steps. However, here are five suggested movements:

1 Stand still with your feet together. Jump forward a few inches with your feet together, then jump back. Clap your hands in front of you each time you jump. Swing your arms and elbows back and away from your body after each clap.

2 Jog lightly in place with your hands loose and elbows close to your sides. Then jog forward, stretching your arms over your head in a V position and looking up.

3 Stand with your legs apart. Stretch your right arm as far as you can to the right, holding it parallel to the floor, without lifting your feet. Stretch from your waist as you extend your arm. Hold the extended position for two counts. Repeat to the left.

4 Take two side steps to the right, ending with your feet together. Then take two steps to the left. Swing both arms forward and then back as you move rhythmically.

5 Stand with your feet together and your arms bent, elbows at a 90-degree angle. Move your right leg forward, keeping your back straight. Push your arms straight out. Bring your right foot back and pull your arms back to the bent position. Repeat, alternating left to right.

These are just a few suggestions; you will surely be able to devise routines of your own. Once you have established a regimen that keeps your heart functioning within the target zone, perform your routine three times a week. If at any time you find that you are breathless or dizzy, or if you have muscle pains after exercising, you are doing too much. Alter your program.

After dancing, cool down for at least five minutes using the suggested strength exercises and flexibility exercises. Then relax completely.

GUIDELINES FOR DANCING

- Wear loose clothing. You may want to invest in a leotard and tights that are especially designed for easy movement. Ballet slippers can be used, but you can just as easily dance in your bare feet or in sneakers.

- Select music that you like. Try to vary the tempos, using slower music early in your routine and working up to a faster pace.

- Many dance books are on the market. Leaf through a few of these books to get ideas for various steps; avoid those that are unduly complex.

- Instead of devising your own routine, you may want to take dance classes. Check the Yellow Pages for a dance school near you. Classes can be expensive. You may want to take one or two formal classes per week and on alternate days do your own dance exercise program.

- Remember, any movement done rhythmically can be a dance movement. Be creative!

Dancing is such an enjoyable method of doing endurance exercises that you may be interested in learning a particular technique or dancing with a group. Many organizations now provide combination dancing and exercise programs; your local YMCA, associations that specialize in folk dancing, or commerical dance centers may have programs that would appeal to you. If you join a dance group and you are concerned about cardiorespiratory improvement, make sure the dancing is vigorous enough so that you'll be exercising within your target zone.

☐ Bicycling

Bicycling is one of the best endurance exercises. It quickly and easily allows you to bring your heart rate up into your target zone, and it's fun.

The only drawbacks to bicycling are the expense of buying the bicycle itself and your dependency on good weather. (But you can get equal benefit from using a stationary bicycle; see below.) Nevertheless, as a vigorous, healthy exercise, few sports surpass bicycling.

A BICYCLING PROGRAM

To get maximum benefit from bicycling, you should ride your bicycle for thirty minutes at least three times a week on nonconsecutive days. For the first five minutes of riding, warm up by riding at a leisurely pace on flat ground. For the next twenty minutes, ride vigorously. Try to ride on hilly terrain, at a fast pace, or using a higher gear. Be sure that your heart is functioning within your target zone. For the last five minutes, bicycle at a leisurely pace.

Alter this program to suit your age and your present condition. Also, be sure to increase your time and the intensity of your riding as you become better conditioned.

GUIDELINES FOR BICYCLING

- Wear loose comfortable clothing. In hot or cold weather, cover your head with a kerchief or hat. This will help protect you from dizziness or heat exhaustion in hot weather and overchilling in cool weather.

- While cycling, relax and lean forward slightly.

- Adjust the height of the seat so that when a pedal is fully depressed, your leg is slightly bent at the knee.

- Always wear bicycle clips if you are riding with loose-fitting pants.

- If you cycle after dark, be sure your bicycle is equipped with lights and reflectors. Wear reflector strips on your clothing as well.

- Check periodically to see that your brakes, horn or bell, wheels, and gear shifts are in good working order.

- Wear a bicycle helmet to protect your head from injury.

- Obey all traffic regulations and rules of the road. Keep to the right. Drive with traffic, not against it. It may be easier for you to see cars if they come toward you, but it is difficult for a driver to see you coming at him, particularly when he is turning. (Fifty percent of the serious bicycle accidents with cars occur at intersections.)

- When driving in traffic, use hand signals to let drivers know you are turning or stopping.

STATIONARY BICYCLES

If the weather is frequently bad where you live or you do not have access to suitable outdoor cycling areas, you may wish to use a stationary bicycle in your home. You can get the same benefits from a stationary bicycle that you can from riding a regular bicycle. Moderate-priced models ($75 to $120) and expensive models ($300 to $400) are equipped with calibrated resistance settings that make it possible to determine your speed and distance. You can then set goals for yourself and practice a regular routine. Low-cost models are usually of limited value since it is difficult to measure and duplicate the amount of resistance needed without calibrated resistance settings.

☐ Indoor exercises

The next three endurance exercises—jogging in place, jumping jacks, and side hops—are all indoor exercises. They have the advantage of being endurance exercises that can be done in a limited space. If you use these exercises as the endurance phase of your program, make sure you include warm-up and cool-down phases as discussed on pages 27–28.

Jogging in place

Purpose
To improve your cardiovascular system and respiratory system as well as the leg muscles.

Starting position
Stand erect with feet a couple of inches apart.

Action
Run in place, lifting your feet 4 to 6 inches off the floor. Hold your arms at your sides at a 90-degree angle.

Note
If you jog indoors, wear gym socks and jog on a rug. If you jog on a hard surface, wear jogging shoes or shoes that cushion your feet.

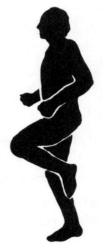

Jumping jacks

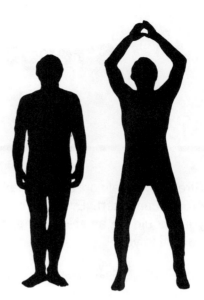

Purpose
To improve your cardiovascular system and respiratory system as well as leg and shoulder muscles.

Starting position
Stand erect with hands at your sides and feet together.

Action
1 Start with a slight jump, spreading feet approximately 2 feet apart while at the same time swinging arms upward until your hands meet over your head.

2 Bring feet together by jumping; at the same time swing arms down to each side. Repeat.

Side hops

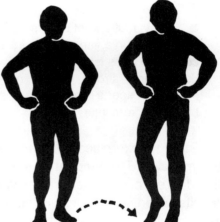

Purpose
To mildly stimulate the cardiovascular and respiratory systems and prepare them for more vigorous exercise.

Starting position
Stand erect with feet together and hands on hips.

Action
1 Hop approximately 12 inches to the left.

2 Hop back to starting position.

3 Repeat steps 1 and 2 to the right side.

> **The preceding set of endurance exercises offers a number of choices. Choose the ones that you like, and change them occasionally for variety.**

CHAPTER 11
Strength exercises

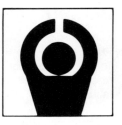

Strength is defined as the maximum amount of force a muscle or muscle group can exert. Even if you are not interested in developing muscles, you should be aware of other reasons why strength exercises can be important to you:

1 As muscles weaken, the structural relationships among parts of the body gradually shift, leading to the aches and pains associated with aging, including back pain. Strong abdominal muscles are especially important to maintain proper alignment of internal organs and to maintain the pelvis in a position that avoids excessive curvature of the lower back. (See Chapter 18, "Lower-Back Pain Prevention and Relief Program.")

2 Strong muscles are firmer and, therefore, more attractive, as is good posture. Looking good is a major reason many people participate in active exercise.

3 Many adults want to take part successfully, and without injuring themselves, in a variety of sports activities. Strong muscles can frequently contribute to better performance while also providing protection from injury. For example, strong muscles in the front of the thighs can contribute to success in sports like tennis and skiing, and at the same time can protect the knees from injury.

Strength exercises must be done fast enough and long enough to tire the muscles. The amount of strength developed is in direct proportion to the degree of overload. The overload principle states that improvement results when the muscle is made to do more than it customarily does. This can be accomplished by adding resistance, by adding repetitions of the exercise, or by speeding up the repetitions. These are called resistance, volume, and speed overload.

☐ Guidelines for strength development

If you use strength exercises to warm up or cool down, do the exercises gently with no attempt to overload the muscles. If you do these exercises to strengthen specific muscles, exercise until you sense some discomfort, but not to the point where you experience pain. If a muscle is to be contracted maximally, the force should be increased gradually over several seconds, held for about 6 seconds, and released gradually to reduce the risk of injury.

Try to balance your program with exercises for the legs, back, arms, and abdomen. You should avoid building strength too unevenly since imbalance in strength among muscle groups makes you more susceptible to injury.

Allow sufficient time between workouts to permit the muscles to recover fully. For calisthenic-type exercises one day is usually sufficient time for recovery; therefore in the beginning, start by exercising three days a week nonconsecutively.

Review these exercises and check back to your "Profile Record" in Chapter 2. Choose exercises that will strengthen particularly weak areas or exercises that look as if they will be enjoyable for you. Do at least two minutes of strength exercises after your endurance training.

STRENGTH EXERCISES	
Abdominal curl	page 62
Half-knee bends	page 63
Graduated pushups	page 64
Weight raiser	page 65

Certain exercises from among the flexibility exercises can also be used to develop strength. These are:

Body twists	page 73
Leg raiser	page 73
Back leg lifts	page 74
Side leg raise (on hands and knees)	page 74
Doorknob leg raiser	page 75

Abdominal curl

Purpose
To strengthen abdomen and lower back.

Starting position
Lie on your back with your legs straight and together and your arms straight against your sides.

Action
1 Slowly bend and lift knees and bring them towards your chest.

2 At the same time, slowly lift your head and back off the floor while sliding your elbows backwards to support you.

3 When your back is fully supported by your elbows (keep your forearms flat on the floor), continue bringing your knees toward your chest as far as possible.

4 Hold this position briefly (one or two seconds), then go back to the original position, slowly lowering legs and back and sliding elbows forward until the original position is reached.

5 Repeat steps 1 through 4 five times.

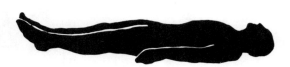

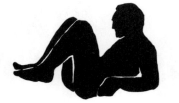

Half-knee bends

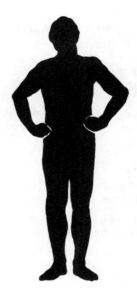

Purpose
To strengthen thighs, calves, hips, buttocks, lower back, ankles, and shoulders.

Starting position
Stand erect with feet spread shoulder-width apart; place hands on hips.

Action
1 Bend knees halfway, bringing heels off ground, while extending arms forward at shoulder level with palms down.

2 Return to starting position.

3 Repeat steps 1 and 2 five times.

Note
Formerly people did this exercise at a full squat, but too many knee injuries resulted—the half-knee bend described here is safer.

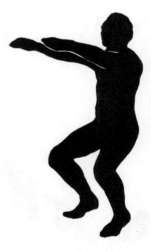

Graduated pushups

Purpose
To strengthen chest, shoulders, upper arms, and upper back.

Starting position
Place palms flat against the surface (wall, chair, or floor). Make sure your arms are straight with elbows locked, your back is straight and rigid, and your legs are straight (unless you are doing variation C).

Action
1 Slowly lower yourself by bending your elbows until nose and chest touch the surface.

2 Slowly push back up and lock elbows again, making sure to keep your back straight and rigid.

3 Repeat steps 1 and 2 five to ten times.

Variations
A Against wall.
B Against table, dresser, chair.
C Against floor, on knees.
D Against floor, knees straight.

Note
Start with the method that is easiest for you.

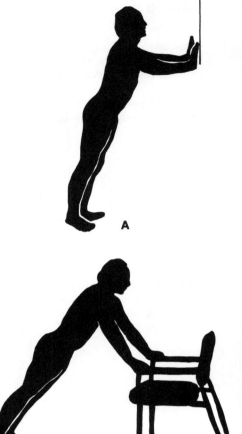

A

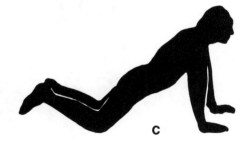

B

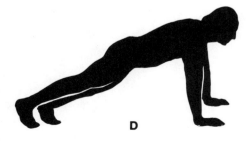

C

D

Weight raiser

Purpose
To strengthen chest, shoulders, and arms.

Starting position
Lie on your back on the floor. Bend knees and place feet flat on the floor, arms extended straight out from the shoulders and resting on the floor.

Place a 2½- to 3-pound weight in each hand. Try using books, 1-quart bottles filled with water and capped, or 2-pound bags of rice.

Action
1 With elbows locked, raise arms until hands meet over your chest.

2 Lower arms to the floor directly behind your head.

3 Raise arms back over your chest.

4 Lower arms to starting position.

5 Repeat steps 1 through 4 five times.

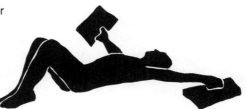

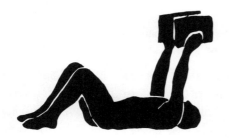

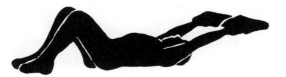

CHAPTER 12

Flexibility exercises

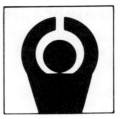

Flexibility can be defined as the range of motion of any given joint. It is extremely important to include flexibility exercises in your program along with endurance and strength exercises. In general, flexible bodies can absorb more stress with less injury. Also, muscles that have been tightened by exercises such as running need to be stretched out again to keep the body in alignment and to avoid injury and muscular aches and pains.

Two types of stretching techniques make up flexibility exercises: the *static* type, in which the stretch is applied gradually, and the *ballistic* type, in which the stretch is applied quickly. Both techniques improve flexibility, but the static type is preferable because it is less likely to result in soreness and injury. In fact, slow-motion limbering may be used to help *relieve* mild soreness.

The following flexibility exercises may be used as warm-up exercises. When used for warming up, they must be done *slowly* and *not* to the limits of your range of motion. When used to stretch the muscles, however, these movements should be done to the limit of your range of motion (but without pain or strain).

Do flexibility exercises after your strength exercises for *at least three minutes*. If you are interested in limbering particular muscles, select the appropriate exercise and do it longer and with greater intensity. For cooling down, do flexibility exercises gently.

Forward and
backward bends

Purpose
To cool down gradually and relax after a workout.

Starting position
Stand erect with feet shoulder-width apart, arms extended in stretched position over your head. Breathe deeply.

Action
1 Exhale slowly while bending knees slightly and bending upper body, arms, and head downward until you are hanging in a loose, relaxed position.

2 When you feel the need for air, begin inhaling while slowly raising your body and arms to the starting position.

3 Bend backward as far as possible.

4 Return to starting position and repeat steps 1 through 3 three times.

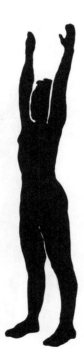
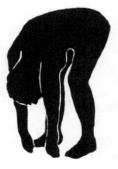

Head rotation

Purpose
To stretch and limber neck and upper back.

Starting position
Stand erect but relaxed, with feet shoulder-width apart and arms behind your back. Look straight ahead.

Action

1 Let your head fall forward and then far to the right in one smooth motion until you can look at the floor behind your right shoulder. Reverse the motion and return to the starting position.

2 Let your head fall forward and to the left in one smooth motion until you can look at the floor behind your left shoulder. Reverse the motion and return to the starting position.

3 Repeat 1 and 2, alternating the motion from right to left.

4 Repeat steps 1 through 3 four times.

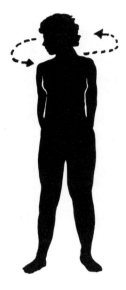

Up and down stretch

Purpose
To stretch muscles of arms, shoulders, chest, and upper back.

Starting position
Stand erect with feet shoulder-width apart and arms hanging loosely at your sides.

Action

1 Raise and stretch arms over your head until wrists touch.

2 Stretch arms in a circle downward until wrists touch in front of your abdomen.

3 Repeat steps 1 and 2 ten to twelve times.

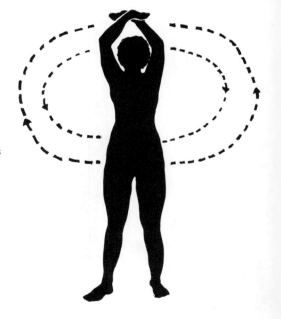

Shoulder-level arm swings

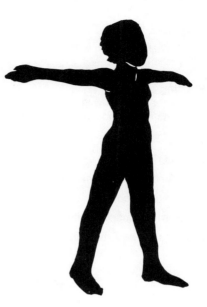

Purpose
To limber shoulders and upper arms.

Starting position
Stand erect with feet shoulder-width apart. Thrust chest out and stretch arms out sideways at shoulder level with palms up.

Action
1 With fingers closed into a fist, swing arms forward, keeping arms straight.

2 As arms come together, open fists and clap your hands gently in front of you.

3 Swing arms slowly back to starting position with chest thrust out and fingers wide open.

4 Repeat steps 1 through 3 five times.

Side bends (one arm raised)

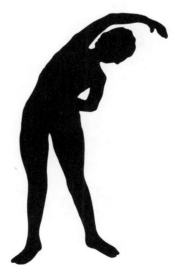

Purpose
To stretch and limber waist, back muscles, vertebrae, and sacroiliac joints.

Starting position
Stand erect with feet slightly wider than shoulder-width apart. Place right arm behind your back and raise your left arm straight above your head.

Action
1 With chest thrust forward, shoulders back, and abdomen tucked in, bend your body to the right until you feel a slight pull at your waist. Hold the position for 4 seconds.

2 Repeat step 1 four times.

3 Reverse position of arms and repeat steps 1 and 2 to the left side.

Alternating leg bends

Purpose
To stretch muscles of legs, hips, waist, buttocks, and lower back.

Starting position
Place feet far apart with legs straight. Place hands on knees and lean forward from the waist.

Action
1 Bend right knee.

2 Return to starting position.

3 Bend left knee.

4 Return to starting position.

5 Repeat steps 1 through 4 four times.

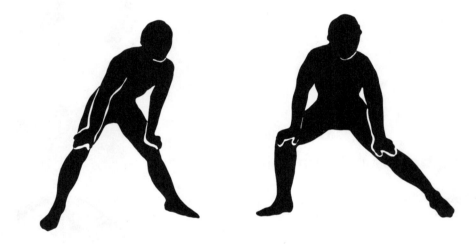

Sitting single-leg raise

Purpose
To stretch muscles of your abdomen, waist, and thighs.

Starting position
Sit on the floor with knees bent and feet flat on the floor. Place your hands on the floor behind you for support. Keep moving your hands farther back until you find a position that is comfortable for you. Keep arms straight and elbows locked.

Action
1 Extend your right leg slowly upward until it is straight.
2 Point your toes as you extend your leg.
3 Lower your right leg smoothly to the starting position.
4 Repeat steps 1 through 3 with the left leg.
5 Repeat steps 1 through 4 four times.

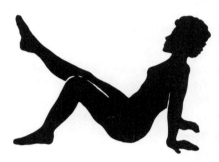

Toe touching

Purpose
To stretch waist and back muscles.

Starting position
Stand erect but relaxed, knees slightly bent. Keep your back straight and let arms hang at your sides.

Action
1 Bend down from the waist until your fingers touch your toes.
2 Bounce very gently up and down two or three times.
3 Return to starting position.
4 Repeat steps 1 through 3 three more times.

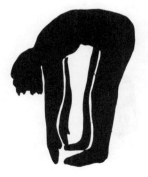

Achilles tendon and calf stretch

Purpose
To stretch calf and Achilles tendon.

Starting position
Stand about 2 feet from a wall with both hands pressed on the wall at shoulder level. (The actual distance you stand from the wall will depend on your height; however, you must be far enough away from the wall to feel a tug in your leg and in the Achilles tendon when you lean forward.) Press heels to the ground.

Action
1 Keeping your knees and hips straight, lean into the wall until you feel a pull behind the knee or leg.

2 Increase the tension gradually.

3 Relax.

4 Repeat steps 1 through 3 four times.

Note
This exercise is especially good for those who use jogging as their endurance exercise.

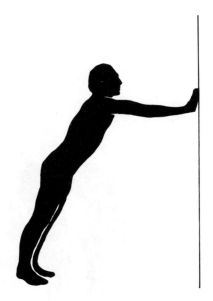

Body twists

Purpose
To stretch muscles in legs, hips, lower back, and waist.

Starting position
Lie on the floor on your back, legs straight, and stretch your arms out sideways straight from your shoulders.

Action
1 Lift one leg straight up.
2 Cross it over your other leg and touch toe to floor.
3 Bring leg back to straight up position.
4 Lower your leg smoothly to original position.
5 Repeat steps 1 through 4 with the other leg. Alternate legs four times.

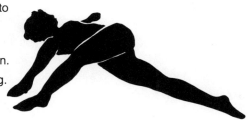

Leg raiser

Purpose
To stretch muscles in your waist, lower back, thighs, and buttocks.

Starting position
Lie on your right side with your body in a straight line; your right arm should be straight and extended under your head. Rest your head on your arm. Place the palm of your left hand on the floor alongside your chest for support. Legs should be straight. Do not roll forward or backward during the exercise.

Action
1 Slowly raise left leg as high as you can. Hold the position for a few seconds. Then bring it down slowly and smoothly.
2 Repeat four times.
3 Reverse position and repeat on your opposite side.

Back leg lifts

Purpose
To limber lower back, buttocks, and thighs.

Starting position
Place a cushion on the floor. Lie face down with hips across the cushion. Fold your arms in front of you and rest your head on your hands. Keep legs straight and feet together.

Action
1 Lift right leg slowly upward, keeping leg straight.

2 When it is as high as you can raise it, hold it raised for four counts.

3 Slowly lower your leg until it is resting on the floor.

4 Repeat steps 1 through 3 with left leg.

5 Alternate legs four times.

Side leg raise (on hands and knees)

Purpose
To stretch thighs, hips, lower back, waist, and buttocks.

Starting position
Get on your hands and knees with arms straight and elbows locked.

Action
1 Extend right leg sideways with leg straight and knee locked.

2 Lower it until the foot almost (but not quite) touches the floor.

3 Raise it back up.

4 Repeat steps 2 and 3 eight times.

5 Bring right leg back to starting position and repeat steps 1 through 4 with your left leg.

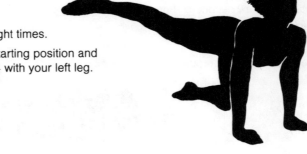

Doorknob leg raiser

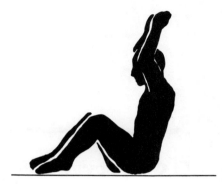

Purpose
To strengthen abdomen, thighs, and arms.

Starting position
Sit tall with your back flat against a firmly closed door. Center the doorknob above your head. Raise your arms above you and grip the doorknob firmly. Bend your knees and keep feet flat on the floor.

Action
1 Raise your feet off the floor several inches.

2 Open and close your legs two or three times.

3 Extend your legs straight out, still keeping them several inches off the floor.

4 Again open and close your legs two or three times.

5 Bring feet back to starting position.

6 Repeat steps 1 through 5 three times.

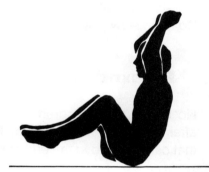

Notes
If lifting both legs at once is too difficult, raise one leg at a time. Remember to keep your back as flat as possible against the door.

This exercise may be difficult for taller people. If you find this is true, do abdominal curls (page 62) to achieve the same benefits.

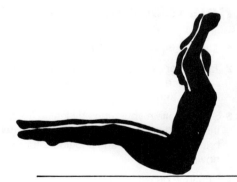

From these activities that promote cardiovascular endurance, muscle strength, and flexibility, choose those exercises best suited to your purposes, those that are most enjoyable to carry out, and those that fit in best with your schedule and environment.

Don't forget, whatever program you choose, to include a cool-down phase.

CHAPTER 13

Cool-down and relaxation

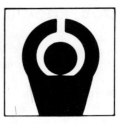

☐ Cool-down

It is imperative that each exercise program have a cool-down period to prepare your body for relaxation and to gradually decrease your heart rate.

Alternate strength and flexibility exercises for a total of five minutes. Do them slowly and without intensity. End with a flexibility exercise.

☐ Relaxation

No matter what program you follow, include a few minutes of relaxation after you have cooled down. The following is a simple relaxation exercise that can be used at the end of your exercise session.

Relaxation exercise

1 Stand normally with your arms at your sides.

2 Take a very slow, deep breath. Your lungs should feel full. Think of yourself as a balloon, inflating and deflating.

3 Slowly deflate your lungs by letting the air out. At the same time, bend forward from your waist, bringing your head and shoulders forward and down.

4 Continue deflation until you are completely bent at the waist, with arms hanging limply and knees slightly bent.

5 Hold this position for two seconds, and when you feel that all the air is out of your lungs, say the word "help" without inhaling any air. This will clear out the last of the stale air in your lungs and prepare them to take in their full capacity again.

6 Reverse this procedure by slowly taking air in
and lifting yourself back to your starting position.
At the end of inhalation, say the word "ease."

7 Repeat this exercise two or three times.

After doing this exercise, you should also take a few minutes to recline comfortably and think pleasant thoughts or listen to music. You may also wish to use one of the more elaborate relaxation techniques suggested in Part 6, such as meditation or massage. When you finish your program with at least a few minutes of relaxation, you should feel completely refreshed, ready to either sleep or begin a new day.

The Health Action Plan exercises in this section provide all the components you need to devise your own program. If you continue to exercise following these guidelines, you will meet your goals and feel better too.

Part 5 and Part 6 include selected special programs that can be used alone or as a supplement to an exercise program.

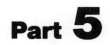

Part 5

Moderate fitness programs

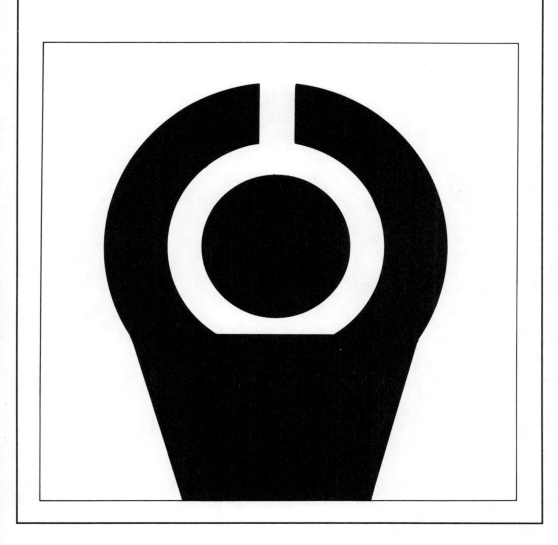

CHAPTER 14
Introduction

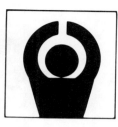

Vigorous activity and exercise may not be appropriate or healthy for everyone. Older people, extremely sedentary people, or those recovering from illness should never plunge into a vigorous exercise program. Although some older and sedentary people may in fact be able to build up their bodies sufficiently to partake in an active program, they should begin slowly.

Many physical changes occur in the body with advancing age. Body weight and heart volume often increase while heart rate and muscle strength usually decline. General metabolism also slows down so that the body requires fewer calories. Bones naturally become more brittle, joints stiff and less flexible.

People who lead extremely sedentary lives and are often overweight and people recovering from illness are apt to be out of shape. Their cardiovascular and respiratory systems are not in top condition. Muscles have become weak and flabby.

These people need a moderate program to slowly recondition their bodies. Two moderate programs are presented here: "A Moderate Exercise Program for Older and Sedentary People" and "A Walking Program." Both programs provide repetitive activity involving the major muscle groups, as well as endurance exercises to improve circulation, provide better support for the spine, and assist in keeping the joints supple. These programs will also help to develop firm supporting muscles that will protect bones and joints from injury. The walking program specifically serves to help increase vigor, make breathing easier, and reduce body fat.

CHAPTER 15
A moderate exercise program for older and sedentary people

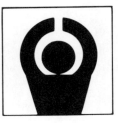

This program is especially designed for older people, for people who have been ill, or for those who have led an extremely sedentary life for a long period of time. In other words, this is a special program for those who are not in condition to partake in a vigorous exercise program, but still want to stay as fit as possible.

Like "The Basic Health Action Plan for Physical Fitness," this program is divided into four parts: a warm-up phase, an endurance phase for cardiovascular development, a cooling-down phase incorporating strength and flexibility exercises, and a relaxation phase. The goal is to improve muscle tone, stimulate circulation, and make joints more flexible. Also, like the basic program, you can select from a number of moderate exercises and construct a plan that suits your particular needs.

It is impossible to dictate absolute time frames for a moderate fitness program because needs can vary greatly. It is, therefore, very important that you pay close attention to your heart rate target zone. Reread Chapter 4, "Heart Conditioning and Your Target Zone," carefully, and make detailed notes on your "Exercise Record," following the sample on p. 37, especially during the first few weeks of exercising. Alter your program as you see fit. Make sure your heart is functioning within its target zone for at least five minutes at first and up to ten minutes as you become more fit. If you find that your heart is functioning below your minimum target zone for your age, increase the amount of time you do your endurance exercise; if your heart is functioning above your maximum target zone rate, reduce activity. Also, take note of your recovery rate. Your heart rate should have returned to normal after ten minutes.

To develop the body and to maintain fitness, begin by doing your program three days a week, on alternate days. Record your progress carefully.

☐ Special note

It is particularly important for older people and people who have been ill to check with a doctor before beginning any exercise program. Have your doctor tell you if you are fit enough to begin this program and be guided by this advice in selecting appropriate exercises.

Over a period of time, you will become progressively more fit. Eventually, you may be fit enough to begin "The Basic Health Action Plan for Physical Fitness." Stay in touch with your body. If you feel you'd like to try the more vigorous program, check with your doctor before you begin.

☐ A few general tips for older and sedentary people

- If you become winded or experience other discomfort while exercising, rest for a while.

- Keep your knees flexed while exercising to avoid strain on your back and joints.

- Exercise at your own pace. You are not competing with anyone.

- Avoid sudden or jerky movements that can cause muscle injuries.

- Proceed slowly and regularly. This is the best way to build strength and stamina.

- Exercise to music or with a companion to make the procedure more enjoyable. (This is good advice for *all* exercise programs.)

☐ Warm-up

It is as important to warm up for a moderate exercise program as it is for a more vigorous exercise routine. Spend at least two minutes warming up. Concentrate on what you are doing by counting the steps you take or by keeping time. Begin to clear your mind of all other matters.

For the first minute, walk in place. Take low or high steps, whichever feels more comfortable. For the second minute, exercise your arms. Swing them back and forth. Relax your shoulders and chest; take deep breaths through your nose and mouth.

Be sure to take a full two minutes to warm up. Rest for a few seconds before you go on.

☐ Endurance exercises

As with any basic fitness program, the endurance exercises are the pivotal part because they are designed so that you will achieve cardiovascular fitness. With a moderate program, you should do your selected exercises for at least five minutes and work up to about ten minutes. It is imperative to exercise within your heart rate target zone. Monitor your heart rate and make sure that you are exercising enough, but not too much.

For this program, we have suggested jogging in place and arm and leg swings as basic endurance exercises. You may also include walking as an endurance exercise. (See Chapter 16, "A Walking Program.") Walk in place or, if the weather permits, take a ten-minute walk outdoors.

Rest for a few seconds before going on.

Jogging in place

Purpose
To improve the functioning capacity of the heart and lungs.

Action
For complete directions for jogging in place, see page 58. For the first week or two, jog by just going onto your toes, alternating feet. As you get into condition, begin to lift your feet off the floor. Be cautious with this exercise. You'll be using muscles that have been dormant, and too much exertion can result in pain.

Note
Always jog on a soft surface such as a rug or carpet. Jogging in bare feet or soft shoes on a hard surface can cause injury to your feet and knees.

Arm and leg swings

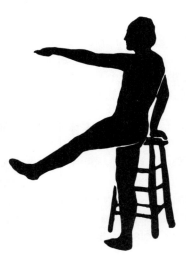

Purpose
To condition hip and shoulder muscles and joints; to stimulate the heart and respiratory rate.

Starting position
With your right hand, grasp the back of a straight chair, the edge of a table, or the top of a stool.

Action
Swing your left arm and leg forward and backward for fifteen to twenty swings. Turn, grasp support with left hand and swing right arm and leg forward and backward fifteen to twenty times.

☐ Strength exercises

A few strength exercises are imperative in any exercise program, even if your goal is not to build huge muscles. Strong muscles, regardless of your age, are necessary for good posture and to protect the bones and joints from injury. Moreover, a strong body is simply more attractive.

If you are older or have been ill or sedentary, do strength exercises gently. Do not attempt to overload your muscles; strength will grow with regular exercise.

In this moderate exercise program, a combination of strength and flexibility exercises is used to aid you in cooling down effectively. For strength, select two or three exercises that you will enjoy doing or that you feel will be particularly beneficial to you. Do these exercises for about two minutes at first. As you become stronger, increase the time and intensity of your strength exercises.

Pushups

Purpose
To build and condition the tricep muscles of the arm and the shoulder muscles.

Action
For complete directions, see "Graduated Pushups," page 64. Begin by doing pushups from the wall. As your strength increases, do pushups from a chair set against the wall. Pushups from the floor are the most difficult. Although you may try them if you wish, you will get adequate effect from the other positions.

Knee bends

Purpose
To condition thigh and calf muscles and arches.

Starting position
Holding the back of a straight chair for support, stand with your knees slightly bent and feet shoulder-width apart. Extend your other arm out to the side.

Action
With a straight chair behind you, squat down until you are in a seated position, *almost* sitting in the chair. Then return to the standing position. (Your heels will lift off the floor as you squat.) Repeat up to fifteen times or until you feel tired.

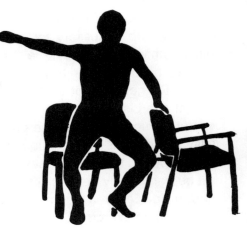

Chair raise

Purpose
To condition the biceps and shoulder muscles.

Starting position
Place the back of a straight chair toward you, the seat away. Stand holding the back of the chair with arms extended straight down, as though it were a set of weights.

Action
Lift chair slowly by bending your arms, then slowly return to position of arms extended. Do not bend your back, although you may round it forward slightly. Repeat five to fifteen times, or until you feel tired.

If the chair is not heavy, lift it straight up in front of you, as far as you feel comfortable. Hold it along the sides of the back—about the level of the seat. Repeat five to fifteen times, or until you feel tired.

Note
If you find lifting a chair difficult or precarious (be sure the seat can't fall out), use a book instead. Use a book heavy enough for the exercise to be effective. A desk dictionary might work well. This variation may also be done sitting down.

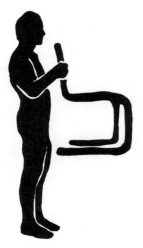

Sit-ups

Purpose

To strengthen abdomen and back muscles.

Starting position

Lie on the floor on your back. Place arms straight at your sides; bend knees so that feet are flat on the floor. Anchor your feet under a piece of heavy furniture or have someone hold your feet down.

Action

Slowly raise your body to a sitting position. Use your elbows for support, if necessary. Slowly lower your body to the original position. Repeat five to twenty times.

Note

You may do this exercise on a bed if you have a hard mattress. Never do sit-ups on a soft mattress; you can strain your back.

If you find this exercise too strenuous at first, try working up in stages. For the first week, just lift your head; for the second week, lift your head and shoulders; for the third week, come halfway up; and finally graduate to a full sit-up.

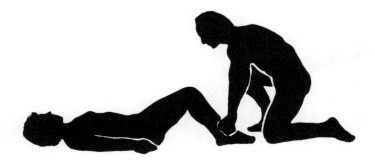

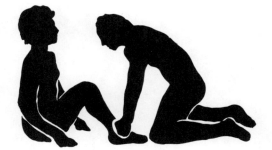

Body twists

Purpose
To strengthen abdomen and back muscles.

Starting position
Lie on the floor on your back, legs straight, and stretch your arms out sideways straight from your shoulders.

Action
Lift your right leg straight up, cross it over your left leg, twisting your body, and touch the floor near your left hand. Bring leg back to straight up position and return to original position. Repeat five to ten times.

Switch legs and repeat body twists with the left leg five to ten times.

Note
You can do this exercise on a bed if you have a very hard mattress. Never do this exercise on a soft mattress. You can strain your back if you do.

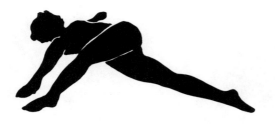

☐ Flexibility exercises

Flexibility or stretching exercises are also an important part of any exercise regimen. In general, flexibility is essential so that your body can absorb stress and ward off injury. Also, after you have been exercising, your muscles will be tight and they need to be limbered.

Flexibility exercises and strength exercises combine to make up the cool-down phase of the moderate exercise program. Select two or three exercises that seem appealing to you. Spend two to three minutes doing flexibility exercises after you have done a few strength exercises.

Arm circles

Purpose
To limber shoulder muscles and joints.

Starting position
Stand erect with feet shoulder-width apart. Stretch arms out straight from the shoulders with elbows locked.

Action
Swing arms in large circles so that the top of the circle is above your head and the bottom is at your waist. Do ten to twenty circles clockwise, then switch and do ten to twenty circles counterclockwise.

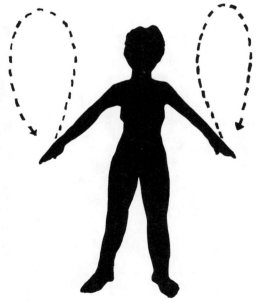

Neck exercises

Purpose
To limber muscles and vertebrae in your neck.

Head bends
Bend your head forward so that your chin touches
your chest. Grasp your hands at the back of your
head. Lift your head *slowly* against the resistance of
your hands until you see the ceiling. Then grasp
your hands against your forehead and press your
head forward. Repeat twice.

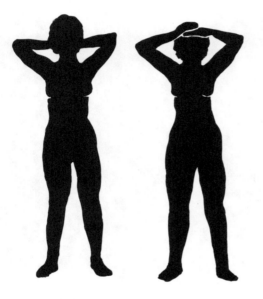

Head rotation
Stand erect with legs apart. Do this exercise slowly
to avoid dizziness.

Roll head downward until you see the floor.
Begin to roll your head to the right and keep turning
until you see the floor over your right shoulder.
Look up to the ceiling.

Roll your head until you can see the floor over
your left shoulder. Keep rotating until you are
actually making a circular motion with your head.

You may feel a "crackle" in your neck as you
do this. This is normal, but do not force your neck
into any painful position. If you get dizzy, stop this
exercise or try making smaller circles.

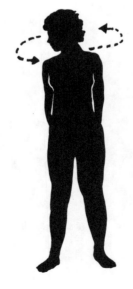

Note
You can do one or the other of these exercises or
combine them.

Side bends (one arm raised)

Purpose
To stretch and limber waist, back muscles, vertebrae, and sacroiliac joints.

Starting position
Stand erect with feet slightly wider than shoulder-width apart. Place your right arm behind your back and raise your left arm straight above your head.

Action
With chest thrust forward, shoulders back, and abdomen tucked in, bend your body to the right until you feel a slight pull at your waist. Hold the position for 4 seconds. Stretch gently to the right eight to ten times. Switch arm positions and bend as far as you can to the left. Stretch gently again eight to ten times.

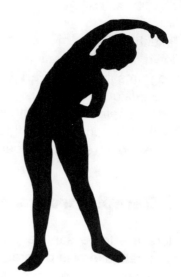

Forward and backward bends

Purpose
To condition back vertebrae and sacroiliac joints.

Starting position
Find your position by standing with your legs far enough apart so that when you bend over your fingertips go below your knees and, if possible, touch the ground. Start with your arms stretched upward and your back arched backward. You may feel more comfortable if your knees are bent slightly.

Action
Bend forward, slowly and gently bringing your arms down so that your fingertips extend below your knees and, if possible, touch the floor. Stretch back upright and arch your back until you feel a stretch. Repeat about five to ten times.

Note
If this exercise makes you feel dizzy, omit it.

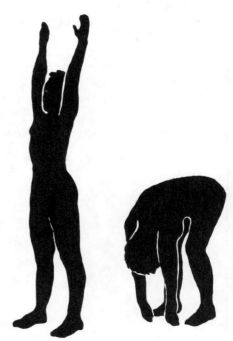

☐ Relaxation

Take three to five minutes to completely relax after you have finished cooling down. Do the relaxation exercise on page 76, select one of the relaxation programs found in Part 6, or simply recline quietly and think pleasant thoughts or listen to music.

After relaxing, you should feel a sense of complete well-being—almost a "high." You will feel free of tension and ready to either start the day refreshed or retire for a sound sleep.

☐ Sample programs

Here are three sample programs to guide you as you devise your own moderate exercise program. Check your "Profile Record" and try to select exercises to condition particular areas of your body that might be weak. Also, be sure to select exercises you will enjoy! Your program should be pleasurable as well as beneficial.

Remember that the time frames are very general. Keep in touch with the response of your body, especially with regard to endurance and your heart rate target zone. Exercise for at least five minutes within your target zone, but don't overdo it, particularly in the beginning.

Exercise three times each week, allowing one day in between each workout for your body to recover. As you become more conditioned, increase your exercise time and the intensity of particular exercises.

SAMPLE PROGRAM 1

Phase	Exercise	Time
Warm-up	Walking in place	2 minutes
Endurance	Jogging in place	3 minutes
	Arm and leg swings	2 minutes
Cool-down:		
Strength	Pushups	1 minute
	Sit-ups	1 minute
Flexibility	Side bends	1 minute
Relaxation	Relaxation exercise	1 minute
	Reclining comfortably	2 minutes
	TOTAL TIME	
	13 minutes	

SAMPLE PROGRAM 2

Phase	Exercise	Time
Warm-up	Walking in place	1 minute
	Arm circles	1 minute
Endurance	Walking outdoors	10 minutes
Cool-down:		
Strength	Knee bends	1 minute
	Chair raise	1 minute
Flexibility	Arm circles	1 minute
	Forward and backward bends	2 minutes
Relaxation	Meditation	5 minutes
	TOTAL TIME	
	22 minutes	

SAMPLE PROGRAM 3

Phase	Exercise	Time
Warm-up	Walking in place	2 minutes
Endurance	Jogging in place	5 minutes
Cool-down:		
Strength	Sit-ups	2 minutes
	Chair raise	1 minute
Flexibility	Neck exercises	1 minute
	Forward and backward bends	1 minute
Relaxation	Relaxation exercise	2 minutes
	Self-massage	3 minutes
	TOTAL TIME	
	17 minutes	

☐ Record keeping

As with "The Basic Health Action Plan for Physical Fitness," it is extremely important for you to keep a record of your progress. See the "Exercise Record" on page 37 and use this form as your guide. Pay particular attention to recording your resting pulse rate, your exercising pulse rate, and your recovery rates. Be sure that you are exercising within your target zone, but not beyond it. Also, watch your recovery rates. If it is taking you too long to recover, you are exercising too vigorously and should cut back.

Finally, keep careful notes on how you feel. Note exercises you particularly enjoy or exercises that result in aches or pains. Revise your program according to your needs and desires.

CHAPTER 16

A walking program

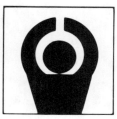

Perhaps the simplest and most convenient activity that can contribute to fitness is walking. This is especially true if you are overweight, out of shape, older, or very inactive. The idea, however, is not to stroll or saunter, but to walk purposefully and to develop over a period of time a good brisk pace (about 3 miles an hour). It is also important to walk daily. An hour a day is suggested.

Walking regularly and vigorously, over progressively longer periods of time, trims the body and strengthens and tones the muscles, especially in the legs. It also keeps the joints more flexible and improves circulation, digestion, and sleep. In addition, it can help with problems of weight control.

Besides being a fine way to prepare for an exercise program, walking is an excellent supplement to such a program. On days when you are unable to do other exercises, a brisk walk can keep you in tone. In fact, as you slowly get into better shape, you will probably have a greater inclination to walk.

Determine the pace and distance you walk by your capacity. In other words, walk as fast and as far as you can while still feeling comfortable. Work toward lengthening the distance you walk and the amount of time you walk. As you get into better shape, you will, of course, be able to walk longer distances in shorter periods of time, so it is important to monitor your progress and periodically expand your program.

☐ A sample walking program

A walking program can help you attain more than one goal. It can improve cardiovascular and respiratory function, increase your energy level, and firm the body by reducing fat.

The following program is a simple, beginning program. Virtually anyone should be able to do it and benefit from it. As you get into better shape, though, you will want and need to increase your pace. Progress gradually, but regularly.

	Exercise	Suggested time
PHASE 1 Warm-up	Walk at an easy pace	5 minutes
PHASE 2 Vigorous walking	Walk at a brisk pace that does not tire you (if you feel breathless, slow down)	10 minutes
PHASE 3 Cool-down	Walk at an easy pace	5 minutes
		TOTAL TIME 20 minutes

PROGRESSION SCHEDULE

The following are three suggested weekly schedules. If you feel you can do even more, don't hesitate to do so.

	Warm-up	**Vigorous walking**	**Cool-down**
WEEK 1	5 minutes	10 minutes (if you can)	5 minutes
WEEK 2	5 minutes	15 minutes	5 minutes
WEEK 3	5 minutes	20 minutes	5 minutes

After the third week, you can choose one of the following:

1 Increase the distance you walk during each session.

2 Walk twenty minutes vigorously *twice* a day.

3 Add exercises to your walking program.

4 Decide to maintain the pace of Week 3 for a while.

EVALUATING YOUR PROGRESS

The best way to evaluate your progress is to listen to your own body. Do you feel refreshed, more relaxed, and less tense after a walking session? Do you find breathing to be easier after walking? As you slowly progress, do you find that in general you are less tired? Do you find that you are less stiff and are suffering fewer aches?

If you keep it up, you will be able to answer "yes" to all of these questions.

MAINTENANCE SCHEDULE

To maintain newfound muscle tone, vigor, and general well-being from walking, you must maintain a regular program. We recommend walking at least three times a week on alternate days—or more, if possible. Aim for at least a thirty-minute program with five minutes of warm-up, twenty minutes of vigorous walking, and five minutes of cool-down. In addition, as you get stronger, you should be covering a greater distance.

RECORD KEEPING

As with other exercise programs, it is helpful to keep a record of your progress. Following the sample on the next pages, record your progress during the first two weeks of your walking program. Continue to keep notes on your progress as the weeks pass. You'll be pleased and perhaps surprised at your development in this moderate exercise program.

GENERAL TIPS ON WALKING

- Wear comfortable, well-supported, low-heeled shoes and absorbent socks.

- Walk as long and as far as you can without discomfort.

- Walk at a brisk pace, and maintain that pace for twenty minutes. You will probably have walked about a mile or at the rate of 3 miles per hour. (Walking a mile in twenty minutes uses up 100 calories.)

- If you find you get tired during your first attempt, slow down, but try to complete the full mile. Be sure to walk at this pace at least three times per week. The key idea is sustained activity—at least three times a week.

- Walking is a noncompetitive exercise geared to your age and weight, so walk at your own pace. Obviously a twenty-year-old can train at a faster rate than a sixty-year-old, yet if each walks for twenty minutes to an hour each day at his or her own pace, each will get the same benefit. Remember, moderate activity for one may be too strenuous for another.

- You may perspire slightly even in cold weather. This is a good sign; it means you are producing a beneficial amount of work for your heart without overdoing it. (Be sure to wear a hat and scarf so that you will not get a chill.)

- Get someone to walk with you. Talking while walking is pleasant and makes the time pass faster, but don't forget to keep up the pace.

- If you walk on hilly terrain, warm up briefly on level ground or on ground that slopes downhill.

A weekly walking record

WEEK 1

	DAY 1	DAY 2	DAY 3*
PHASE 1 **Warm-up** Walk easily	✓ 5 min.	✓ 5 min.	✓ 5 min.
PHASE 2 **Conditioning** Walk at a brisk pace	✓ 10 min.	✓ 10 min.	✓ 10 min.
PHASE 3 **Cool-down** Walk easily	✓ 5 min.	✓ 5 min.	✓ 5 min.

WEEK 2

	DAY 1	DAY 2	DAY 3*
PHASE 1 **Warm-up** Walk easily	✓ 5 min.	✓ 5 min.	✓ 5 min.
PHASE 2 **Conditioning** Walk at a brisk pace	✓ 15 min.	✓ 15 min.	✓ 10 min.
PHASE 3 **Cool-down** Walk easily	✓ 5 min.	✓ 5 min.	✓ 5 min.

*For the rest of the days of the week, continue in the same format.

Part 6

Special programs

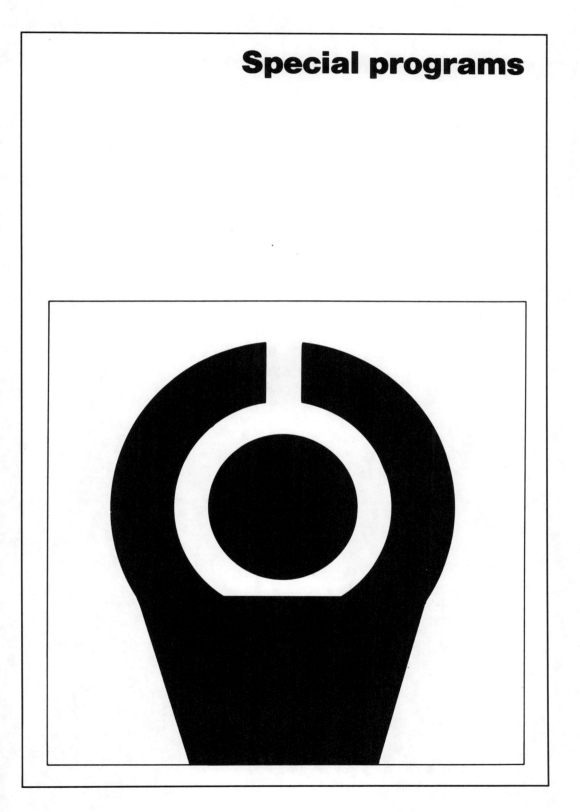

CHAPTER 17

Programs for relaxation and relief of tension

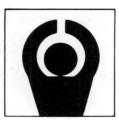

True fatigue is caused by intense physical activity or prolonged mental activity. Different people have different capacities for physical activity, and a proper exercise program can increase that capacity.

"False fatigue," a condition of tiredness just like that which results from overwork, can be caused by tension, boredom, and lack of sufficient physical activity. Its symptoms—tiredness, irritability, apathy—are the same as those of true fatigue.

The relaxation programs that follow are tested methods that can help you eliminate "false fatigue." In addition, any one or a combination of these programs will have the following results: relaxation, relief of muscular and psychological tension, and increased energy. The yoga-type exercises will also give you increased flexibility and improved muscle tone. These programs can easily be supplemented or alternated with any of the previously described activities.

You have five choices:

- Relaxation techniques
- Isometrics
- Yoga-type exercises
- Meditation
- Massage

On days that you carry out these activities try to evaluate how effective they are for you. Do they help reduce tension? Do they relax you? Do you feel somewhat refreshed afterward? By answering these questions you will be able to select the activities that do you the most good. Do not be afraid to experiment and try other activities. In general, deep breathing, brief periods of pleasant meditation, and walking have been found to be very helpful to most people suffering from "false fatigue." However, do not expect instantaneous results. Like everything else, you must learn these techniques well in order to benefit.

☐ Selected relaxation techniques

■ Set your alarm clock a little earlier than usual. Eat a light, leisurely breakfast while you listen to pleasant music.

■ Take a brisk walk—even if it's for only five minutes. Breathe deeply, observe your surroundings—shop windows, trees, people, the color of the sky.

■ Practice keeping your face—especially your lips and brow—relaxed (as if you were just about to smile).

■ Do three or four minutes of warm-up exercises a few times a day or whenever you feel tense.

■ Sit with your hands on your thighs, elbows at the sides, and back straight but not touching the back of your chair. Inhale deeply to the count of seven, pause for a second, and exhale. Repeat five or six times. Do this several times a day and whenever you feel tense (even when you are stalled in traffic or waiting for an appointment).

■ Sit comfortably, close your eyes, and concentrate on something you find attractive, beautiful, or appealing. Try to eliminate any other thoughts. Breathe deeply and rhythmically. Do this for a few minutes whenever you feel tense, bored, or tired.

☐ Isometric exercises

If you have trouble relaxing, isometric exercises can help you unwind or fall asleep. The principle of isometrics is to first tense your muscles and then slowly relax them. Do isometrics in bed or lying on the floor. Breathe easily and rhythmically while doing them; try not to hold your breath or breathe rapidly.

1 Lie flat on your back in bed with your arms at your sides and your legs out straight. Let all muscles relax.

2 Curl your toes just as far as possible until you start to feel discomfort. Slowly, passively, let your toes relax until they are completely relaxed.

3 Point your toes forward as far as you can. Hold them there until you start to feel uncomfortable. Slowly relax, letting them return to their normal position.

4 Push your heels down hard, until you can feel the muscles tighten up your leg and into your buttocks. Push until the muscles feel a little bit uncomfortable, then slowly and progressively let the muscles relax until your legs feel completely relaxed.

5 Pointing your feet away from each other, try to touch the bed or floor with your little toes. Keep your heels on the bed or floor. Tighten all the muscles that are in this area strongly until it feels uncomfortable. Hold for a second, then slowly let the muscles relax until you feel no tension at all.

6   Rotate the legs inward and try to touch the bed or floor with your big toes. Contract these muscles until you feel slight discomfort, then let the legs relax.

7   Put your feet together and push your legs and your heels together as hard as you can. Hold this position for a few seconds, then let your legs relax slowly.

8   Squeeze your hands to make a fist. Tighten the fists, using all the muscles you can, as hard as you can. Relax them slowly until your hand is relaxed.

9   Sit in any comfortable position on the floor. Place your palms on the floor and push your arms down into the floor. Try to lift your body with your arms straight at your sides. Push hard, then relax slowly.

10   Turn your hands over so the backs of your hands are on the floor. Push again, the way you did before, as hard as you can. Relax slowly.

11   Close your eyes just as tightly as you can, hold it, then relax slowly.

12   Close your jaws together just as tightly as you can. Relax slowly.

13   Raise your eyebrows and wrinkle your forehead hard, then relax slowly.

14   Lie on your back on the floor or bed, pushing the back of your head against the surface just as hard as you can. Keep your neck straight, using your arms and your heels to keep your back flat. Relax slowly.

The isometric method—tightening and then relaxing muscles—can be used whenever you feel tense and is a good office exercise.

□ Yoga-type exercises

Yoga is a Sanskrit word meaning union. It is part of ancient Hindu philosophy and advocates a union of physical and mental disciplines.

Yoga doesn't build muscles, but rather alternately compresses and stretches them. This not only has a relaxing effect but also results in increased flexibility of the muscles and joints. The many different yoga postures also work to strengthen muscles and improve muscle tone.

MEDITATION

An important aspect of yoga that can be used by anyone is meditation, which is recommended before carrying out any of the movements and postures. Even if you do not attempt the simple yoga exercises that follow, you may find that the meditation episode will refresh and relax you.

Assume a simple sitting ("lotus") position, in which the ankles are crossed in front of you and drawn in as far as possible. A half-lotus position with one ankle drawn in under the thigh may be easier at first. Keep your body erect, your eyelids lowered (but with your eyes open), and rest your hands on your knees. Now close your eyes and fix your mind on a pleasurable thought. With practice you should be able to clear your mind of extraneous thoughts. It sometimes helps to repeat words that give you a good feeling (beauty, softness, love) or words that conjure up images that you find attractive (mountains, clouds, flowers, seashore). Any pleasant sound may be repeated.

This period of meditation should last for a minimum of five minutes and preferably for ten to twenty minutes. Many persons find that this peaceful interlude of rest in a pleasurable state is highly restorative and relieves physical and emotional tension. (For more details on meditation, see "Meditation," page 109.)

YOGA-TYPE EXERCISES

Below are a few simple yoga activities you may wish to try after your meditation. They should be done in a quiet setting with enough space to stretch your limbs. Wear comfortable clothing to allow for freedom of movement. Use a mat or folded blanket.

Full and rhythmic breathing

Sit in the cross-legged posture or "lotus" position. Slowly exhale through your nose. (All breathing should be done through the nose.) While exhaling, contract your abdomen until your lungs are completely empty. Then *slowly* inhale while pushing out the abdomen. While still inhaling, slightly contract your abdomen and expand your chest as much as you can. Continue to inhale and slowly raise your shoulders as high as you can. Hold your breath with your shoulders raised for about three seconds. Then slowly begin to exhale deeply while contracting your abdomen and allowing your body to relax. Continue inhaling and exhaling in this manner for a few minutes.

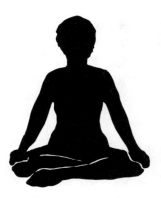

"Cobra" position

The "cobra" position releases tension in the spine. Lie on your stomach with your forehead on the mat and your arms at your sides. Let all your muscles relax. Now bring your hands up and place them beneath your shoulders with the fingers of each hand touching, pointing toward each other at right angles to the shoulders. Very slowly raise your head and bend it backwards.

Push against the floor with your hands and slowly raise your trunk. At the completion of this movement your head should be well back with your eyes looking upward. The elbows should be still slightly bent, your spine arched, and your legs relaxed. Hold this position for about five seconds. Now slowly reverse the movements and lower your body until you are once again in the starting position. Pause briefly and repeat once. Then rest your cheek on the mat and allow yourself to go completely limp.

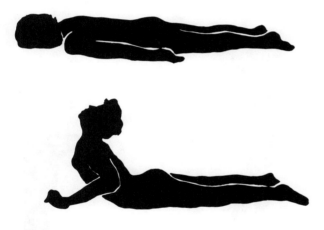

Chest expansion

The chest expansion releases tension in the shoulders. Stand with your heels together and arms at sides. Slowly bring your hands up until they touch your chest. Now slowly stretch your arms straight in front of you as far as possible. You should feel your elbows stretching. Slowly bring the arms back behind you as high as you can. Lower your arms slightly so that you can interlace your fingers. Now raise your arms as high as possible without straining. Do not bend forward. Gently bend your head backward several inches, looking up. Keep arms as high as you can and your knees straight. Hold this position for a few seconds. Now very slowly bend forward so that your head is hanging down. Raise the arms (with your fingers still interlaced) up behind the back. Your neck should be limp and you should be looking toward your knees. Slowly straighten up, pause for a moment, and repeat the movements.

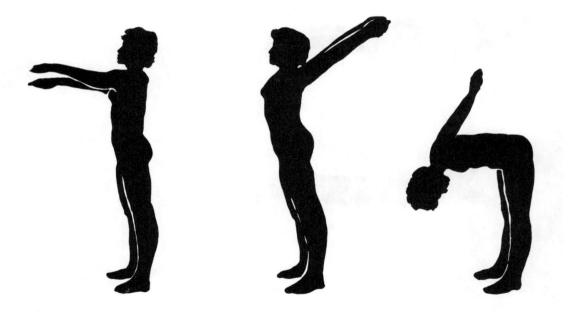

Neck exercise

The neck exercise releases tension in the neck. Sit on the mat in a comfortable position. Close your eyes. Carry out motions very slowly. Lower your head so that your chin rests on your chest; hold for ten seconds. Roll your head to the extreme left; hold for ten seconds. Roll your head back as far as you can; hold for ten seconds. Roll your head to the extreme right; hold for ten seconds. Roll your head forward again so that your chin rests on your chest and hold for ten seconds. Repeat these movements in the opposite direction, going first to the right.

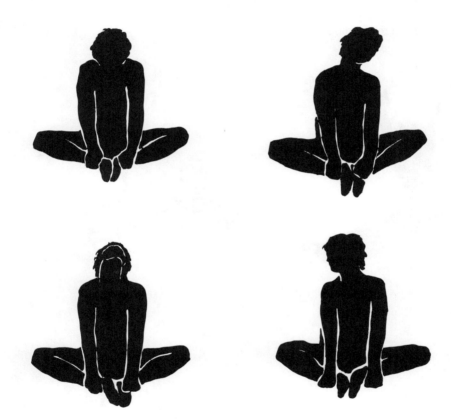

Alternate leg stretch

The alternate leg stretch releases tension in the legs. Do this exercise slowly. Sit with your legs stretched in front of you. Take hold of your right foot and place the right heel and sole so that they rest against (not under) the left thigh. Raise your arms overhead and lean backward several inches. With your head back, look up. Lean forward with arms outstretched. Take a firm grip on your left calf (if this is difficult, bend your knee slightly). Pull against the elbows and aim your forehead at your knee; hold for ten seconds. Slowly straighten up and stretch arms above head, looking up. Repeat the stretch; then switch legs so that your right leg is outstretched and repeat the stretch twice.

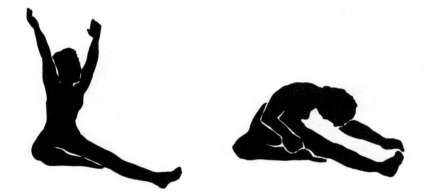

If you are particularly interested in yoga and wish to know more about it, look for a program at the local Y. There are also many books that describe and illustrate this discipline.

□ Meditation

Why is meditation included in a book on physical fitness? The answer has been given by the athletes of ancient Rome—*"Mens sana in corpore sano"*—a sound mind in a sound body.

No matter what exercise program you choose, whatever physical fitness goal you select, you will achieve it with greater satisfaction if you are free of anxiety and relieved of psychological stress. In this regard both meditation and physical exercise supplement one another in creating a sense of well-being. If you jog, swim, or do calisthenics in a state of mental agitation, you will not be able to obtain either the maximum satisfaction or the maximum benefit from your efforts.

Meditation can help reduce stress. Although meditation is often surrounded by mystery, all meditation techniques follow similar concepts that can be learned and practiced easily without previous training.

Meditation can be used with any exercise program you choose, or you may omit it if you feel it is not for you, but don't underestimate it or ignore it. You should be aware that it is a valid, time-proven way of establishing a calm, tranquil psychological state without using medications, drugs, or alcohol.

WHAT CAN MEDITATION ACHIEVE FOR YOU?

- Psychologically it can help you feel calm, free of anxiety, and mentally refreshed. It can create a pleasant, and in some cases heightened sense of well-being. It can provide the same kind of euphoria that you experience after exercise but without fatigue. It will put you in an agreeable emotional mood.

- Physiologically, meditation induces a hypometabolic state such as is found when sleeping, but meditation is not sleeping. You are in control of your consciousness. (In this respect meditation also differs from hypnosis.)

- It changes the brain waves as determined by the electroencephalograph, so that alpha waves predominate. Alpha waves are associated with a resting mental state; they disappear with agitation.

- When you meditate, your heart rate, rate of breathing, and blood pressure decrease.

- Although meditation is not a substitute for sleep, meditation can be a prelude to refreshing sleep and can eliminate the need for tranquilizers and sedatives. For some people this may be its most important benefit.

BASIC REQUIREMENTS FOR MEDITATION

Some basic conditions must be fulfilled in meditation, and you must experiment to determine how you can work these conditions into your lifestyle.

The basic requirements for meditation are:

1 *A quiet place* where you can go at approximately the same time each day, a place free of distractions where you cannot be reached by telephone. This may not be easy to find. You may have a room where you can be by yourself, but freedom from distracting sounds is difficult if you live in an urban area. If necessary use earplugs during meditation. You can purchase them in any drugstore or you can use cotton soaked in heavy mineral oil or Vaseline. (Be sure to wring out the excess mineral oil before using the cotton plugs.)

2 *Get into a comfortable position.* Loosen your clothes, but you do not have to change into special clothing. A comfortable position in a chair or seated on the floor with your head held erect is satisfactory. The cross-legged yoga position called the "lotus" is favored by many, but it is not essential. A lying-down position is used by some people, but this is too conducive to sleep and sleep is not the objective. Meditation is best done sitting with the back straight, head erect, hands on the thighs or on armrests.

3 *Make a conscious effort to relax the body and clear the mind.* We are often not aware that our brows are furrowed, our teeth clenched, our shoulders hunched, our abdominal muscles tight. Think about your major muscle groups and consciously relax them. Then relax your mind. Do not let any external thoughts, current problems, or chronic anxieties intrude. Close your mind to them, and assume a deliberately unagitated state. It may be difficult to do at first, but with practice you will be able to achieve this condition with a minimum of effort. The ability to keep external thoughts out of your mind is an essential precondition for meditation.

4 *Turn your awareness to your breathing.* Breathing is a completely involuntary activity, a function of the autonomic nervous system. For the purpose of meditation you do not have to control it, just be aware of it. Concentrate on the process of inhaling-exhaling, considering yourself a detached but intensely interested observer. Focusing on this vital body function will assist you in developing the proper frame of mind. It will keep the mental door shut on outside thoughts. At this point your thoughts are turned inward and are concentrating on a vital body function.

5 *Dwell on a repetitive sound, image, or idea.* Dwelling on something is necessary to maintain the next step in actual meditation, when you, your entire nervous system, your thought processes, your voluntary and involuntary nervous system are free of external or self-imposed pressure.

While this is occurring you are conscious and aware but your thoughts are turned inward. The feeling is similar to what you might experience when gliding silently underwater in a pool—quiet, serene, tranquil, and yet aware of a pleasurable sensation.

Concentrate on inhaling and exhaling, silently repeating a word or sound with the process, or repeating, for example, the number "one" or any other number, with each breath. Another autonomic function that is repetitive and can be focused on in the meditative state is the pulse. If you are sitting absolutely quietly you can feel the blood pulsating through your body and you can silently repeat a number or sound in harmony with your pulse beat.

An alternative focal point for your thoughts is an *imagined image,* such as ocean waves, rowing a boat, a flower, or a portion of your body, such as the center of your forehead. Silently repeat the name of the object as you visualize it.

A *repeated sound* may be used instead of an image. Tennyson repeated his own name during meditation and you may wish to use your name. You may also wish to use a part of a prayer or poem, or a pleasant sound. You may find added enjoyment by incorporating a harmonious thought, phrase, or word in your meditation. In the formal systems of meditation, particularly those originating in Eastern religions, you are given a word, a "mantra" (the Sanskrit word for a chant), to use as a repetitive sound. In other systems a number or sequence of numbers is used. There is nothing magic in this. You may choose your own pleasant soothing sound or repeat a number. Experiment until you find what works best for you. All of the above techniques are preferably done with the eyes closed.

Another repetitive action is concentrating on a *real image*. This may be a single object in your room, a flower, a religious object, or a picture. One technique is to use a lighted candle, fixing on it with the eyes open, then closing the eyes and maintaining the image. If you are having difficulty maintaining the image or outside thoughts intrude, open your eyes to reinforce the image of the lighted candle and then close them again.

HOW MUCH TIME SHOULD BE SPENT MEDITATING?

At first, meditate five minutes per day. Gradually increase the time to twenty or thirty minutes daily. Try to meditate at the same time each day, such as in the morning, after work, or before you go to bed.

HOW DO YOU KNOW IF YOU ARE SUCCESSFULLY MEDITATING?

First, don't try too hard; do not carry over your daily drive-to-achieve attitude into meditation. If you can sit still for five to thirty minutes and direct all your thoughts inward, allowing no distractions or conscious thoughts of everyday living, *you are meditating*. The more frequently you do it, the more effective it will be.

Meditate every day. Meditating is something that requires education and gets better with practice, but is quickly lost through disuse. Even if you do it for only a few moments a day, practice. It is a great psychological tool to have available to you when you need it. However, if you stop for a long period of time it will take special effort to reeducate yourself.

A FEW ADDITIONAL THOUGHTS

- Setting an alarm clock for the time you put aside for meditation may be helpful at the beginning. (This will eliminate the need to keep checking the time.) Most people follow the wisdom of their bodies. With training, you will complete the meditation in the twenty or thirty minutes that is the average amount of time most people meditate.

- Some people use background music while they meditate. You can buy tapes and records to assist in meditation—even a tape of a heart beating, which is advocated by one system of meditation. However, in general, it is advisable not to have external stimuli of any kind. Turning inward and getting in tune with the autonomic nervous system does not require any external stimuli.

- A few moments of stretching or walking about after meditation, a kind of cool-down, is advisable as a transition back to normal activity. You will not feel sleepy or foggy as you sometimes do when you wake up from a nap.

☐ **Massage**

Massage makes you feel good; it has a relaxing effect. This is the universal reaction of people of all cultures, and it is an observation made throughout recorded history. Massage goes by many names and there are an infinite number of variations, but basically this is what it accomplishes:

- Massage relaxes tense muscles.

- Massage increases the circulation in the areas massaged by friction, heat, and pressure. It causes the blood vessels to dilate and also mechanically assists in venous and lymphatic circulation.

- It has a tranquilizing effect. Stroking soothes a child or animal; it works for adults, too.

- At the completion of massage most people feel refreshed and invigorated.

Some things massage will *not* do:

- It will not make your muscles stronger (although it will decrease fatigue).
- It will not lead to weight reduction.
- It will not remove fat deposits in areas massaged.

THE FOUR BASIC MASSAGE MANEUVERS

1 *Gentle massage (effleurage):* This is accomplished by light stroking motions, little pressure, and has a skin effect only. There should not be enough pressure applied to feel the muscles.

2 *Deep massage (souflage):* A stroking motion with pressure, using the fingertips, heel, or palm of the whole hand. One should feel the muscles ripple beneath the touch. The amount of pressure used is variable. The subject will tell you if more or less pressure is desirable.

3 *Compression (patrissage):* These are deep kneading or compression motions. For example, two hands are used to encircle and compress an arm or leg while a gliding, firm stroke is used. Deep compression is always directed upward toward the heart to assist the circulation. The returning stroke is gentle. On the back and shoulders, roll muscles between the thumb and fingers or beneath the palm of the hand.

4 *Percussion (tapotement):* This is accomplished with a tapping or hacking motion; it can be done with repeated tapping of the fingertips or quick up-and-down motions of the outer edges of the hands. This action is suitable for large muscle groups but should never be done over the abdomen, heart, or breasts.

Beyond these basic motions, there are a large number of special maneuvers devised by professionals or used in special systems of massage, such as knuckle motions, cupping strokes, pulling and pushing, pressure-point systems (such as Shiatsu), and Rolfing (a very vigorous technique of connective tissue manipulation). These are often combined with motions of the extremities and joints for an endless variety of maneuvers. These specialized systems should be left to professional practitioners.

BEFORE YOU START MASSAGE

1 *Work on a firm surface.* A bed is usually not satisfactory, but if you have a firm mattress it may be used. A waist-high table is best, but this usually will not be available in the home. The best substitute is to have the subject lie on a few blankets on the floor.

2 *Use oil, powder, or rubbing alcohol.* These are important adjuncts to the massage. They are placed on the portion of the body just before the massage of that area begins. The oils most frequently used are baby oil or light mineral oil. Powder can be used but is not as good in overcoming friction and can create a dusty atmosphere. Rubbing alcohol is less satisfactory in most instances and should be used only when one desires to create warmth from a slight irritant effect on the skin. As the alcohol evaporates, a great deal of friction and warmth occurs. Use it sparingly, and be careful not to splash it in the eyes or on the genitals. Warm the oil or alcohol first by running the container under hot water for a few minutes before using it.

3 *It is important for the subject to cooperate during the massage.* The mind should be clear; the subject should be listening to music, or better still, focusing on the portion of the body being massaged in a conscious effort to relax the muscles and avoid tensing up against the massaging hands. The cardinal rule for massage is: if it doesn't feel good, if it makes you uncomfortable or self-conscious, do not do it.

HOW TO DO THE MASSAGE

Keep in mind you are not a professional and are not trying to be one. You are helping a spouse or friend to relax, decrease muscle tension, and induce a feeling of well-being.

The best way to learn massage is to experience it yourself at the hands of a professional. Go to a health club or a local Y. Attend the first session to convince yourself of the value of the massage experience. Attend two or three more sessions to observe how it is done. It would be best if your spouse or friend went, too, as you could learn together and later learn from one another.

As you experience the massage from the professional, concentrate on the main strokes. Every professional will have his or her own set of special maneuvers that you would have difficulty trying to duplicate. Do not make it complicated; it doesn't have to be. Use your common sense.

Keep your object in mind: to relax major muscle groups. First, divide the body into five zones:

- Head and neck
- Back
- Legs
- Arms
- Chest and abdomen

Talk over what you are going to do with the subject so that you are in agreement. If he or she wishes any portion of the body omitted, do so. If he or she wishes any portion of the body to remain covered, do so. An atmosphere of confidence and harmony must be established.

The order in which the massage is carried out is not of great importance. Try to develop a mutually satisfying routine. The time for total body massage by a professional will be forty-five minutes to an hour. As a nonprofessional you will wear out before your subject calls it quits. It is good exercise for you, but you will probably tire after thirty minutes. Try to time your efforts so that you spend five or six minutes on each of the five areas.

As you learn from the professional, note his or her actions in the five major areas and adapt them for your own use.

THE MASSAGE

1 *Head and Neck.* A good first motion is a soothing, superficial circular stroke on the forehead and temples, using very little oil. Then proceed to a raking fingertip motion through the scalp, varying the pressure and the rapidity of movement (no additional oil is needed for the scalp), and proceed with deeper finger pressure on the sides and back of the neck. To relax the neck muscles, proceed along the outer portion of the neck, sliding up behind the ear to the temples, forehead, and front of the scalp with moderate pressure. Light circular stroking of the face and submandibular— below the jaw—region is optional. It can be omitted for the purposes of the massage-relaxation, unless the subject feels that this is an area where a great deal of tension is centered.

2 *Back.* The head and neck areas and the back are probably the most important areas for massage, as these are the sites of the greatest muscular tension. Also, it is massage of these regions that gives the deepest sense of comfort. Take long, deep strokes in one direction and superficial strokes in the other. Vary your touch from fingertip to palm to heel of the hand, run your fingertips on either side of the spine, but leave the spine itself alone. Grasp the flanks between your thumb and fingers and feel the muscles ripple beneath your grasp. Do the same for the upper border of the trapezius muscles, the flat triangular muscles behind the neck and shoulders. If you prefer you may include the shoulder muscles with the massage of the head and neck region. For additional pressure when massaging the lumbar (lower back) region, place one hand on top of the other and lean into the deep stroke with your weight. It will be less tiring for you. Your subject will tell you if it feels good or not and you can adjust the pressure accordingly. Similarly, experiment with tapping, hacking, or kneading motions on the muscles of the back.

3/4 *Legs/Arms.* A similar combination of strokes for the arms and legs may be used as described above, using both hands for one extremity at a time. It is usually easier to massage the arms and legs when the subject is lying on his or her back. Also, for massage of the thigh and calf muscles, it is advantageous to have the leg bent at the knee. The arm can be massaged lying in any position away from the body. You may wish to grasp the arm between your own arm and chest while working on the upper portion with both hands. There are several motions that are particularly suitable for the extremities. *Compression* or *drainage* is one. Here the arm or leg is encased with both hands and compressed while pushing up toward the trunk, as if draining fluid from the arm or leg. Another is *wringing*. This is a massage variation of the Indian burn, done with oil. It is not painful, but invigorating. Third is *rolling*, or placing the arm or leg between the flats of the hands at right angles to the length of the extremity and simultaneously thrusting each hand in opposite directions so the muscles of the extremity roll between your hands. When massaging the arms or legs, never place them in an awkward or uncomfortable position. Do not exert pressure on any joints. Despite what you read about methods of massage, never try to manipulate or "crack" joints.

5 *Chest and Abdomen.* The chest and abdomen are not protected with the heavy musculature that one finds on the back. The ribs are just beneath the skin and the heart beats against the chest wall. The organs of the abdomen are also less protected from the front than they are from the back. Thus for massage, strokes to the chest and abdomen should not be as vigorous as for other portions of the body. A good starting move is to stand above your subject and grasp the sides of the chest between your thumbs and hands for a moderately firm to-and-fro motion down the flanks. The pectorals of the upper chest and shoulder girdle can be firmly massaged with the fingertips in small circles or to-and-fro motions. For the abdomen itself, a light, followed by a moderately firm, circular motion may be used. A particularly good stroke for the abdomen is to-and-fro pulling. Standing at either side of the subject, with a half-bend of the fingertips and a hand on each flank, rake back and forth across the abdomen with the hands passing each other in opposite directions. This motion can be started at the hips and then can proceed to the upper abdomen. Stop as you reach the lower portion of the chest. The knees may be bent or straight for these strokes.

Complete the massage with long, gentle, full-body strokes. Chances are the subject will be glowing and relaxed and you will be aching and sweating, so you take the shower first.

A professional masseur would perform many more maneuvers and include the face, hands, feet, and buttocks. Additional techniques can be learned as you gain confidence in your ability.

SELF-MASSAGE

It is remarkable how much relaxation and invigoration you can achieve by self-massage. It is also remarkable to discover how much work it is.

You can, with little difficulty, massage the head and neck area, the face, your arms and legs, chest and abdomen, and lower back.

You can carry out self-massage on the floor, in a bathtub, or in a shower. However, if you are in a bath or shower, do it sitting or reclining in the tub, or sitting on a stool in the shower. Do not attempt self-massage when standing on a wet surface. You will be inviting an accident.

In a bath or shower try massage with a *loofah* sponge or a mildly abrasive mitt, which you can purchase in a drugstore.

A mechanical device that some barbers still use is the electrical vibrator. It is your hand that actually does the vibrating; the vibrator is strapped to the back of your hand. Never use this when you are wet or in the water. It does save a lot of wear and tear on your muscles, but you can achieve the same effect without it.

A whirlpool bath or needle shower is another variation on the massage theme. Here it is the thrust or ripples of water that do the massage. The heat helps in relaxation.

Whether you prefer isometrics, yoga, meditation, or massage, it is important that a special time for relaxation be incorporated into everyday life. This may require a special determination on your part. Modern society does not make this easy, so planning for exercise and relaxation time is the only way. After only a short period of time most people who follow relaxation programs wonder how they got along without them.

CHAPTER 18

Lower-back pain prevention and relief program

Millions of Americans suffer from lower-back pain. The causes are various; damaged vertebrae, ruptured discs, arthritis, and other chronic disorders are frequently the source of the pain. If you have recurrent pain, it is important to have it checked by a physician.

Back pain may also result from tension, stooping for prolonged periods, strain from lifting objects improperly or from sudden forceful back motions, or sleeping on a mattress that is too soft. Think about your daily habits and stresses and consider whether or not one of these may be causing your problem.

If you discover that your backache is not a result of disease, injury, or one of the other underlying causes, it is likely to be due to weak muscles in your lower back and abdomen. In fact, four out of five backaches result from weak muscles. What's more, not only is backache a product of such weakness, but poor posture—itself a producer of backache—also comes from weak muscles. It's an endless cycle.

☐ Testing your abdominal and back muscles

The following four exercises will give you an indication of just how strong (or how weak) your back and abdominal muscles are. Try each exercise. If you find that you are unable to do them, you can be sure that your muscles need strengthening.

1 Lie on your back on the floor with your hands behind your neck and have someone hold your feet down. Slowly curl up into a sitting position, keeping your knees straight.

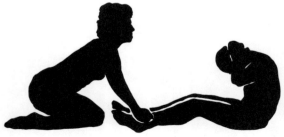

2 Lie on your back on the floor with your knees bent, your feet flat on the floor, and your heels as close to your buttocks as possible. Place your hands behind your neck. Have someone hold your feet down. Curl up slowly into a sitting position.

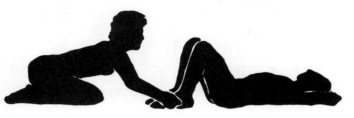

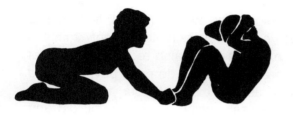

3 Lie on your abdomen on the floor. Place a pillow under your hips and place your hands behind your neck. Have someone hold your feet down. Try to raise your chin and chest off the floor and hold that position for ten seconds.

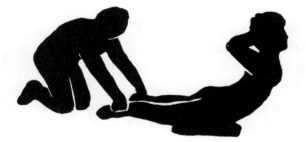

4 Lie on the floor on your abdomen. Place a pillow under your hips. Have someone hold your shoulders down. Keeping your knees straight, raise both legs as high as you can and hold that position for ten seconds.

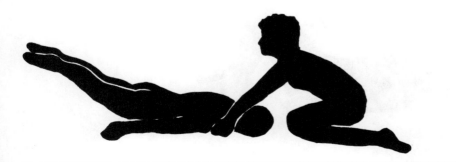

☐ A program for preventing or correcting lower-back pain

If you find that you can't do the preceding exercises, or do them with great difficulty and straining, your muscles are weak. The following program, when undertaken each day, is designed to:

- Strengthen lower-back muscles and abdominal muscles.
- Eliminate lower-back pain and generally prevent back problems.
- Improve posture.

This program has three phases: warm-up, conditioning (or corrective) exercises, and cool-down. You should spend approximately five minutes each warming up and cooling down and approximately twenty minutes doing a combination of corrective exercises. It is also recommended that you keep a record of the number of exercises you do each day, following the sample on page 124. This way, as you evaluate your improvement, you will have a detailed record of precisely which exercises you did and the amount of time you spent working out. Most of us do not have to suffer from lower-back pain; you can provide your own relief by following this program.

☐ The exercises

1 Lie on your back, arms at sides, palms down, knees flexed, and feet flat on the floor. Breathe slowly and deeply through the nose and exhale slowly through the lips. Attempt to relax muscles before starting exercises.

2 Lie on your back, arms at sides, palms down, knees flexed, and feet flat on the floor. Tighten buttocks, draw in belly and keep lower back flat against the floor. Hold position for five seconds, then relax.

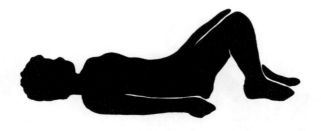

3 Lie on back with knees drawn toward chest and hands clasped around knees. Press shoulders flat against the floor. Pull knees tightly against the chest with arms and raise forehead to touch knees. Hold position for five seconds, then relax.

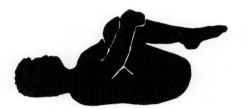

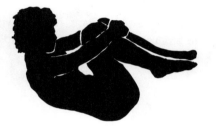

4 Lie on your back and place hands, palms down, under buttocks. Place feet flat on the floor with knees flexed. Tilt the pelvis slightly upward off the floor, press the small of the back down against the floor, and hold for five seconds, then relax.

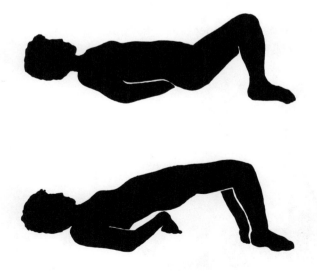

5 Sit on the floor, legs extended forward. Hold abdomen in and try to touch toes with fingers. Use a rocking motion to aid stretching.

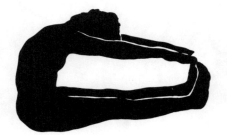

6 Sit on the floor with your legs stretched out in front of you, head down toward your chest as far as it will go. Then relax your back, lift your head, and flex each knee alternately.

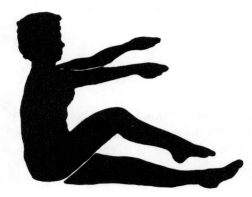

7 Lie on your back and place cushion under hips. Rest your hands behind your head. Lift legs up alternately, keeping knees straight and toes pointed. Relax between lifts.

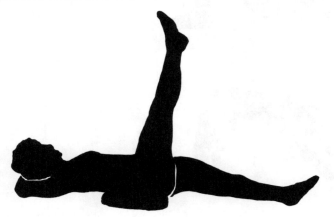

ALTERNATE EXERCISES

Substitute either or both of these exercises if you prefer them to any of the above.

8   Lie flat on your back. Holding left leg between the ankle and knee, pull knee toward shoulder as high as you can. Repeat with right leg.

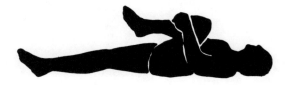

9   Lie flat on your back. Raise legs slightly off floor, holding for one or two seconds. Stretch legs and point toes forward.

LOWER-BACK PAIN PREVENTION AND RELIEF PROGRAM

	Suggested repetitions
PHASE 1 WARM-UP	
Exercise #1	5 times gradually increase to 10 times
PHASE 2 CORRECTIVE EXERCISES	
Exercise #2	start by doing 3 times gradually increase to 10 times
Exercise #3	start by doing 3 times gradually increase to 10 times
Exercise #4	start by doing 3 times gradually increase to 10 times
Exercise #5	start by doing 3 times gradually increase to 10 times
PHASE 3 COOL-DOWN	
Exercise #6	start by doing 3 times gradually increase to 10 times
Exercise #7	start by doing 3 times gradually increase to 10 times

A sample record
LOWER-BACK PAIN PREVENTION
AND RELIEF PROGRAM

PHASE 1

	DAY 1	DAY 2	DAY 3
WARM-UP			
Exercise # 1	✓ 5 times	✓	✓

PHASE 2

	DAY 1	DAY 2	DAY 3
CONDITIONING			
Exercise # 2	✓ 3 times	3 times	4 times
Exercise # 3	✓ 3 times	3 times	4 times
Exercise # 4	✓ 3 times	3 times	4 times
Exercise # 5	✓ 3 times	3 times	4 times

PHASE 3

	DAY 1	DAY 2	DAY 3
COOL-DOWN			
Exercise # 6	✓ 3 times	3 times	4 times
Exercise # 7	✓ 3 times	3 times	4 times

☐ Tips on posture and lower-back care

- Avoid standing in one position for a prolonged period. Hips tend to sag forward after you stand for a long time, and this places a strain on the lower back. To relieve the strain while doing various standing tasks (working at a table, washing, or ironing), flex one hip by placing a foot on a stool, step, or railing.

- Always bend your knees when leaning forward, lifting, or lowering any object.

- Avoid lying flat on your back without flexing the knees. When reclining, place a pillow under the knees to keep the back flat.

- When sitting, keep your knees on the same level as, or slightly higher than, the hips. When driving, be sure the seat is close enough to the pedals so that your legs do not have to be fully extended while working the gas and brake pedals.

- Avoid positions in which your neck and head are thrust forward with the chin tilted up such as watching a sporting contest or sitting in the front row of a movie theater.

- Good posture contributes to your health and appearance. When you are standing, your weight should be equally distributed on both feet. Stand ''tall''—with your body slightly stretched upward without strain.

- When you are sitting, it is important to sit well back in the chair to obtain maximum spine comfort and relaxation. There should be no space between the back of the hips and the chair.

- If you wake up with pain in your lower back, it is usually the result of sleeping on your stomach on a too-soft mattress. If you sleep on your stomach, you should have a pillow under your lower legs so the knees and hips will be more flexed.

- Make sure that your mattress is sufficiently firm. Keep the lower back placed firmly against the mattress.

- When stooping and lifting, always squat, bend at the knees, and keep your back straight. If you lift with your arms by bending your back and failing to squat, you will place an undue strain on the lower-back muscles.

☐ Evaluating your progress

Now that you have begun a program for back care and are familiar with the causes of back problems, check through the following list.

- Has my posture improved? Do I carry myself "tall" as I walk? Do I hold my stomach flat and my shoulders back?

- Do I shift position if I have to stand for a long period of time?

- If I work at a desk, do I stretch and bend at least once an hour to reduce pressure on my spine?

- Am I careful to bend my knees and keep my back straight before lifting an object?

- Do I get at least twenty minutes of activity a day exercising the large muscles of the trunk? Do I walk briskly, climb stairs, exercise regularly?

- Have I checked my mattress to make sure it is firm?

- Do I feel less strain in my back?

Your answers to these questions will tell you whether or not this program is working for you. After a month of following the program, if you are still experiencing back pain or if you are not sure of your progress, perhaps you should contact a physician to make sure you have no hidden reasons for your discomfort.

For most, however, this program will serve both to relieve back pain and to prevent it from recurring.

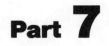

A few final thoughts

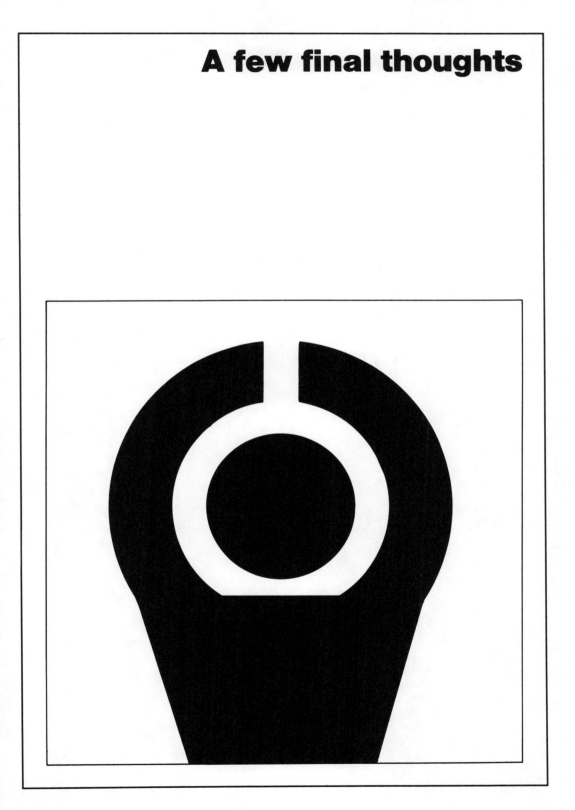

CHAPTER 19
Final thoughts on exercising

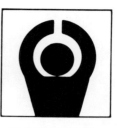

A beginner's total exercise program should not be too vigorous. If you experience extreme soreness or discomfort when you start your program, lower the intensity of your exercises. Try out each exercise briefly the first time. Familiarize yourself with it, then slowly work it into your program.

Any exercise program should be done a minimum of three days per week, allowing one day in between sessions for your body to get used to the added stress. Set the days and times in advance and try to keep to your routine.

Once you find a comfortable pace, stick to it for three sessions. If you feel your program is too easy or too hard, change it slightly the next week. Pay close attention to your heart rate and keep in touch with how you truly feel.

Keep your record-keeping notebook in a convenient place and keep it up-to-date. It is a good idea to enter your feelings, attitudes, thoughts, and perceptions on the chart each time you exercise. Also note your resting heart rate, your exercise rate, and your recovery rates. These are the best clues to whether or not you are exercising adequately and to your ultimate benefit.

If you exercise for a full thirty minutes (build up to this level gradually within your target zone), three times per week, you should be assured of an adequate level of fitness. Advance at your own pace, and take care not to overexert yourself. Remember: if your heart rate remains in the target zone for twenty minutes, you are getting a good workout.

CHAPTER 20
Exercise and your appearance

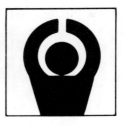

Many people begin to exercise for the purpose of losing weight and improving their bodies. What few people realize is that it takes an enormous amount of exercise to actually *lose* weight. Although any exercise program will firm and tone muscles (which does make for a more attractive body), the simple fact is that you must *eat less as well as exercise* to see a substantial weight loss.

For the purpose of comparison, here are the approximate number of calories expended per minute for various activities. These figures can vary depending upon a person's weight and sex, but as you can see, exercise alone will generally not be enough to control weight. You must also cut calories.

CALORIE/ACTIVITY TABLE

Activity	Calories per minute
Sitting or reclining	1–1½
Standing	2–2½
Walking slowly	2½–3
Calisthenics	3–7
Walking briskly	4–5
Bicycling	6–8
Swimming	9–11
Jogging	10–13
Cross country skiing	15–17
Running or jumping rope	19–20

☐ Tips on appearance

- Losing 1 pound of fat requires "spending" 3,500 calories. You can "spend" 300 calories a day by walking briskly for one hour.

- Moderate exercise before meals tends to diminish appetite.

- Exercise training will normalize the relationship between lean body mass and fat. When a reduction diet is combined with exercise, you will lose both weight and flabby fat.

- To reduce *total body fat,* do exercises—such as jumping rope, bicycling, walking briskly, or swimming—for a minimum of twenty minutes at least three times a week.

- Exercise gives you a glow and a sense of well-being that are as attractive as a sleek body.

A trim and toned body is both healthy and attractive. Check the weight chart on the next page and decide what your weight should be. If you are overweight, combine dieting with your exercise program until you reach your desired goal.

Weight chart of persons twenty years and older

MEN

Height (without shoes)	Weight (without clothing) Normal range	Obesity level*
5'3"	118–141	169
5'4"	122–145	174
5'5"	126–149	179
5'6"	130–155	186
5'7"	134–161	193
5'8"	139–166	199
5'9"	143–170	204
5'10"	147–174	209
5'11"	150–178	214
6'0"	154–183	220
6'1"	158–188	226
6'2"	162–192	230
6'3"	165–195	234

WOMEN

Height	Normal range	Obesity level
5'0"	100–118	142
5'1"	104–121	145
5'2"	107–125	150
5'3"	110–128	154
5'4"	113–132	158
5'5"	116–135	162
5'6"	120–139	167
5'7"	123–142	170
5'8"	126–146	175
5'9"	130–151	181
5'10"	133–156	187
5'11"	137–161	193
6'0"	141–166	199

*A weight above 20% of upper normal is generally considered an obesity level.
Adapted from: U.S. Department of Agriculture, Home and Garden Bulletin No. 74.

CHAPTER 21

A few more tips on exercising

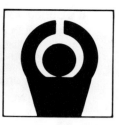

While developing the Health Action Plan, *Physical Fitness,* we worked with many people. Some had exercised for years, some had been thinking about starting a program, some had exercised in the past but had stopped, and some were exercising but were unsure of what gains had been made. We want to share some of their feelings and observations with you and also provide you with some additional advice. Take from these tips and suggestions the ones that seem right for you.

- Exercise with a neighbor, friend, spouse, children. Even the dog can go on a walking or jogging program with you.

- Light competition works for some.

- Change your exercises occasionally to give yourself some variety.

- Exercise to music. (See "Dancing," page 55).

- Exercise before bed if you have trouble sleeping.

- Counteract boredom with gratification. Set a prize for yourself for achieving.

- Do not get upset with yourself if you miss your exercises once in a while.

- You have to keep some sort of record.

- Try alternate programs if one does not work for you.

- Gym equipment is unnecessary. Rely on yourself.

- Tap your own sense of vanity.

- Different people need different programs.

- Put physical fitness into your life-style, your daily activities.

- Keep the program simple.

- Gradual progression is vitally important for two reasons: you will reduce your chance of injury, and you will get satisfaction from advancing to higher levels.

- Do not be discouraged if the benefits are not immediate. It takes regular, long-term effort.

- During your exercise routine, take a break whenever you want to. You are not in competition.

- Rank your goals in order of importance to you.

- Decide on a few long-term goals. Once a short-term goal (such as losing weight) is reached, people tend to stop exercising. Remember, don't lose sight of your ultimate goals. Any exercise program must be continuous.

- Take a close look at your body a few weeks after you have started exercising. You will begin to see a positive change, and this will serve as reinforcement.

- People of all ages can exercise—and benefit from exercise.

- Learn to recognize the difference between moderation and strain.

- Organize your program so that it fits easily into your daily life. It is easier to keep the habit if you exercise at the same time each day.

- Do warm-up activities each session to ready the heart, muscles, joints, and circulation for endurance training and to avoid injury.

- Cool down afterwards. Gradually reduce the intensity of exercise until it reaches a very low level before you stop. (For example, after jogging, walk for a few minutes.) This prevents the blood from pooling in the lower extremities, which can lead to dizziness or light-headedness.

- Allow ten minutes after cool-down before showering. Take a warm shower. *A hot or cold shower can dangerously affect your blood pressure.*

- Avoid extensive or vigorous outdoor exercise or activity when the weather gets hot, especially when there is high humidity. Prolonged strenuous exercise under these conditions can cause dehydration and dangerous elevation in body temperature.

- Wait an hour after a meal before exercising *vigorously* to avoid cramping or nausea. (A leisurely walk after eating is beneficial.)

- If you stop exercising for a while—even a week or two—start at a lower level and gradually work your way up again.

- The ability to perform exercises can vary from day to day even without the influence of illness. If you find yourself tiring early, take frequent short breaks (ten- to thirty-second rest periods) during your training.

- Alcohol and exercise do not mix. Alcohol dilates the blood vessels, diverting blood away from the muscles, where the blood's oxygen is needed most.

- Smoking elevates the heart rate, lowers the oxygen-carrying capacity of the blood, reduces the flow of blood to the muscles and the heart, and reduces breathing efficiency.

- To be physically fit at forty-five is not the same as being physically fit at twenty-five. It is unrealistic to think you can compete with a youngster, but you can be as fit as possible for your age.

After reading the Health Action Plan, *Physical Fitness,* getting in touch with your particular needs and desires concerning exercise, and devising a program that suits them, you have only one task left—to make your personalized program a permanent part of your life-style.

Exercising and getting yourself into good physical condition should be satisfying for you. Using guidelines and advice from this book, you should have been able to put together a program that will work for you. Best of all, it will be a program that will bring you better health and a fine sense of well-being.